Brain Informatics and Health

Informatics-enabled studies are transforming brain science. New methodologies enhance human interpretive powers when dealing with big data sets increasingly derived from advanced neuro-imaging technologies, including fMRI, PET, MEG, EEG and fNIRS, as well as from other sources like eye-tracking and from wearable, portable, micro and nano devices. New experimental methods, such as in toto imaging, deep tissue imaging, opto-genetics and dense-electrode recording are generating massive amounts of brain data at very fine spatial and temporal resolutions. These technologies allow measuring, modeling, managing and mining of multiple forms of big brain data. Brain informatics & health related techniques for analyzing all the data will help achieve a better understanding of human thought, memory, learning, decision-making, emotion, consciousness and social behaviors. These methods also assist in building brain-inspired, human-level wisdom-computing paradigms and technologies, improving the treatment efficacy of mental health and brain disorders.

The Brain Informatics and Health (BIH) book series addresses the computational, cognitive, physiological, biological, physical, ecological and social perspectives of brain informatics as well as topics relating to brain health, mental health and well-being. It also welcomes emerging information technologies, including but not limited to Internet of Things (IoT), cloud computing, big data analytics and interactive knowledge discovery related to brain research. The BIH book series also encourages submissions that explore how advanced computing technologies are applied to and make a difference in various large-scale brain studies and their applications.

The series serves as a central source of reference for brain informatics and computational brain studies. The series aims to publish thorough and cohesive overviews on specific topics in brain informatics and health, as well as works that are larger in scope than survey articles and that will contain more detailed background information. The series also provides a single point of coverage of advanced and timely topics and a forum for topics that may not have reached a level of maturity to warrant a comprehensive textbook.

More information about this series at http://www.springer.com/series/15148

Shui-Hua Wang · Yu-Dong Zhang
Zhengchao Dong · Preetha Phillips

Pathological Brain Detection

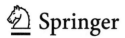 Springer

Shui-Hua Wang
School of Computer Science
    and Technology
Henan Polytechnic University
Jiaozuo, Henan
China

and

School of Electronics Science
    and Engineering
Nanjing University
Nanjing, Jiangsu
China

Yu-Dong Zhang
Department of Informatics
University of Leicester
Leicester
UK

and

School of Computer Science
    and Technology
Henan Polytechnic University
Jiaozuo, Henan
China

Zhengchao Dong
Translational Imaging Division & MRI Unit,
    New York State Psychiatric Institute
Columbia University Medical Center
New York, NY
USA

Preetha Phillips
Shepherd University
Shepherdstown, WV
USA

and

West Virginia School of Osteopathic
    Medicine
St. Lewisburg, WV
USA

ISSN 2367-1742   ISSN 2367-1750 (electronic)
Brain Informatics and Health
ISBN 978-981-13-3834-2   ISBN 978-981-10-4026-9 (eBook)
https://doi.org/10.1007/978-981-10-4026-9

This Springer imprint is published by the registered company Springer Nature Singapore Pte Ltd.
The registered company address is: 152 Beach Road, #21-01/04 Gateway East, Singapore 189721, Singapore

Preface

Machine learning is a prosperous research field in computer science. It has evolved from an initial expert system to a system demonstrating deep-learning techniques. In 2016 the best known breaking news in this field was that AlphaGo, developed by Google, beat the world champion, Lee Sedol, in a Go match in Seoul. This drove the burning enthusiasm of scholars to apply machine learning to other important fields. This book describes the application of machine learning to radiology.

Currently, radiologists and neuroradiologists face the challenge of detecting lesions both rapidly and accurately. Lesions of various diseases in their prodromal phase are not easy to detect with human eyes. However, computers can easily distinguish a slight change in brain's structure. The ability to distinguish a slight gray-level difference can be pivotal in making an accurate and reliable diagnosis.

This book summarizes the latest advances in pathological brain detection using machine-learning approaches. It presents state-of-the-art computer algorithms, which can help perform automatic medical diagnoses in the brain.

This book is for undergraduate and graduate students in the field of computer science. It may also be useful to engineers, scientists, neuroradiologists, and researchers who are interested in pathological brain detection.

This book is organized in the following manner. Chapter 1 provides the basics of pathological brain detection. In this chapter various brain diseases are categorized into four main types.

Chapter 2 introduces neuroimaging modality from a historical view. Pneumoencephalography, cerebral angiography, computerized tomography, positron emission tomography, and single photon emission computerized tomography are all described in this chapter. There is a specific emphasis given to magnetic resonance imaging.

Chapter 3 presents standard image preprocessing techniques, including image denoising, skull stripping, slice selection, spatial and intensity normalization, and image enhancement—subtleties essential to pathological brain detection procedures.

The next six chapters are the basic components of a standard computer-aided diagnosis system. Chapter 4 shows how to extract features from brain images. Chapter 5 describes multiscale and multiresolution features. Chapter 6 introduces wavelet families and variants. Chapter 7 expatiates dimensionality reduction techniques. Chapter 8 compares the latest classifiers. Chapter 9 covers the latest optimization techniques used to train classifiers. All six chapters form a canonical procedure of developing a smart diagnostic system. Each individual chapter is a description of the background reviews of corresponding methods, and introduces and compares related state-of-the-art methods.

Chapter 10 compares current state-of-the-art pathological brain detection systems. Their shortcomings are analyzed to suggest the possible direction of future research. Finally, Chap. 11 shows deep-learning technique results for cerebral microbleeds. The convolutional neural network is found to give better results than an autoencoder and traditional computer vision–based methods.

The four contributors of this book are Dr. Shui-Hua Wang, Prof. Yu-Dong Zhang, Prof. Zhengchao Dong, and Dr. Preetha Phillips. The four authors have a long history of cooperation over the past 10 years. The team has published over 100 peer-reviewed papers in famous international journals. We hope this book might benefit your study and work.

Jiaozuo/Nanjing, China   Shui-Hua Wang
Leicester, UK/Jiaozuo, China   Yu-Dong Zhang
New York, USA   Zhengchao Dong
Shepherdstown/St. Lewisburg, USA   Preetha Phillips

Acknowledgements

This book would not have been possible without the contributions of many people.

We would like to thank those people who commented on the proposal and helped to organize its structure: Shuai Liu, Xing-Xing Zhou, Guang-Shuai Zhang, and Zhu-Qing Jiao.

We appreciate those people who provided constructive feedback on the content of the book: Carlo Cattani, Xiao-Jun Yang, and Liang-Xiu Han.

We are indebted to those who allowed us to reproduce images, figures, or data from their publications. We indicate their contributions in the figure captions throughout the text.

We are grateful to Henan Polytechnic University, Nanjing University, and Department of Informatics at University of Leicester for providing office space, so that we could finish this book. We also thank Matlab software, by which the most of our signal and image processing tasks can be done using one simple command.

Some pictures were downloaded from the "Bing" search engine which were "free to modify, share, and use commercially," and from "Google" search engine which were "labelled for reuse with modification." We would like to acknowledge the authors of these images.

This book is also supported by following foundations:

1. Natural Science Foundation of China (61602250, 51407095, 61503188).
2. Natural Science Foundation of Jiangsu Province (BK20150983, BK20150982, BK20151548, BK20150973).
3. National Key Research and Development Plan (2017YFB1103202).
4. Henan Key Research and Development Project (182102310629).
5. Jiangsu Key Laboratory of 3D Printing Equipment and Manufacturing (BM2013006).
6. Program of Natural Science Research of Jiangsu Higher Education Institutions (16KJB520025, 15KJB470010, 15KJB510018, 15KJB510016, 13KJB460011, 14KJB480004, 14KJB520021).
7. Key Supporting Science and Technology Program (Industry) of Jiangsu Province (BE2012201, BE2013012-2, BE2014009-3).

8. Special Funds for Scientific and Technological Achievement Transformation Project in Jiangsu Province (BA2013058).
9. Open Project Program of the State Key Lab of CAD&CG, Zhejiang University (A1616).
10. Open Fund of the Key Laboratory of Symbolic Computation and Knowledge Engineering of the Ministry of Education, Jilin University (93K172016K17).
11. Open Fund of the Key Laboratory of Statistical Information Technology and Data Mining, State Statistics Bureau (SDL201608).
12. Open Fund of Guangxi Key Laboratory of Manufacturing System & Advanced Manufacturing Technology (17-259-05-011K).
13. Open Research Fund of the Hunan Provincial Key Laboratory of Network Investigational Technology (2016WLZC013).
14. Open Research Fund of the Key Laboratory of Network Crime Investigation of Hunan Provincial Colleges (2015HNWLFZ058).
15. Open Fund of the Fujian Provincial Key Laboratory of Data Intensive Computing (BD201607).
16. Open Program of the Jiangsu Key Laboratory of 3D Printing Equipment and Manufacturing (3DL201602).
17. Open fund of the Jiangsu Key Laboratory of Advanced Manufacturing Technology (HGAMTL1601 and HGAMTL-1703).
18. Open fund of the Key Laboratory of Guangxi High Schools Complex System and Computational Intelligence (2016CSCI01).
19. Key Laboratory of Measurement and Control of Complex Systems of Engineering, Southeast University, Ministry of Education (MCCSE2017A02).
20. College start up funding at Leicester (P202RE803).

Contents

Acronyms

ABC	Artificial bee colony
ACO	Ant colony optimization
AD	Alzheimer's disease
AE	Autoencoder
AF	Activation function
AFNI	Analysis of functional neuroImages
AI	Artificial intelligence
AIS	Artificial immune system
ASP	Algorithm-specific parameter
BBB	Blood–brain barrier
BBO	Biogeography-based optimization
BD	Bhattacharyya distance
BER	Bayes error rate
BET	Brain extraction tool
BF	Bilateral filter
BFGS	Broyden fletcher goldfarb shannon
BGS	Boltzmann–Gibbs–Shannon
BOLD	Blood oxygen level dependent
BP	Backpropagation
CAD	Computer-aided diagnosis
CART	Classification and regression tree
CBF	Cerebral blood flow
CCP	Common controlling parameter
CDF	Cumulative distribution function
CJD	Creutzfeldt–Jakob disease
CLAHE	Contrast-limited adaptive histogram equalization
CMB	Cerebral microbleed
CNN	Convolutional neural network
CSA	Clonal selection algorithm
CSF	Cerebrospinal fluid

CSI	Chemical shift imaging
CT	Computerized tomography
CWT	Continuous wavelet transform
DAE	Denoising autoencoder
DAG	Directed acyclic graph
db	Daubechies (wavelet family)
DCA	Dendritic cell algorithm
DCT	Discrete cosine transform
DE	Differential evolution
DFRFT	Discrete fractional Fourier transform
DFT	Discrete Fourier transform
DNN	Deep neural network
DR	Dimensionality reduction
DST	Discrete sine transform
DT	Decision tree
DTCWT	Dual-tree complex wavelet transform
DTI	Diffusion tensor imaging
DWT	Discrete wavelet transform
EEG	Electroencephalogram
EELM	Evolutionary extreme learning machine
ELM	Extreme learning machine
EM	Expectation–maximization
EP	Evolutionary programming
ERM	Empirical risk minimization
ES	Evolution strategy
FA	Firefly algorithm
FDG	Fludeoxyglucose
FE	Frequency encoding
FFT	Fast Fourier transform
FLIRT	FMRIB's linear image registration tool
FMF	Fuzzy membership function
fMRI	Functional magnetic resonance imaging
FMRIB	Oxford Centre for Functional MRI of the Brain
FNIRT	FMRIB's nonlinear image registration tool
FNN	Feed-forward neural network
FRFT	Fractional Fourier transform
FSL	FMRIB's software library
FSVM	Fuzzy support vector machine
FT	Fourier transform
GA	Genetic algorithm
GEPSVM	Generalized eigenvalue proximal support vector machine
GLCM	Gray-level co-occurrence matrix
GM	Gray matter
GP	Genetic programming
GS	Grid search

GSO	Glowworm swarm optimization
GTB	Gradient tree boosting
HC	Healthy control
HE	Histogram equalization
HIV	Human immunodeficiency virus
HMI	Hu moment invariant
HPF	High-pass filter
HSI	Habitat suitability index
ICV	Inter-class variance
IDFT	Inverse discrete Fourier transform
IELM	Incremental extreme learning machine
IG	Information gain
INA	Immune network algorithm
kFCV	k-fold cross validation
kNN	k-nearest neighbor
KPCA	Kernel principal component analysis
LCDG	Linear combination of discrete Gaussians
LOOCV	Leave-one-out cross validation
LOSI	Logistic sigmoid
LPF	Low-pass filter
LPOCV	Leave-p-out cross validation
LRC	Linear regression classifier
LReLU	Leaky rectified linear unit
LSE	Least-squares estimation
MARS	Microbleed anatomical rating scale
MCCV	Monte Carlo cross validation
MD	Mahalanobis distance
MGRF	Markov–Gibbs random field
MIP	Maximum intensity project
MLP	Multilayer perceptron
MNI	Montreal Neurological Institute
MR	Magnetic resonance
MRA	Magnetic resonance angiography
MRI	Magnetic resonance imaging
MRSI	Magnetic resonance spectroscopic imaging
MRST	Multiple radial symmetry transform
MSE	Mean squared error
MWV	Max-wins-voting
NBC	Naive Bayes classifier
NLM	Non-local means
NPSVM	Non-parallel support vector machine
NSA	Negative selection algorithm
ONN	One-nearest neighbor
OPELM	Optimally pruned extreme learning machine
OSELM	Online sequential extreme learning machine

PBD	Pathological brain detection
PC	Principal component
PCA	Principal component analysis
PDF	Probability density function
PE	Phase encoding
PEG	Pneumoencephalography
PET	Positron emission tomography
PKPCA	Polynomial kernel principal component analysis
PNN	Probabilistic neural network
PPCA	Probabilistic principal component analysis
PR	Pattern recognition
PSO	Particle swarm optimization
PZM	Pseudo Zernike moment
PZP	Pseudo Zernike polynomial
QMF	Quadrature mirror filter
QP	Quadratic programming
RAP	Rank-based average pooling
RBF	Radial basis function
RBFNN	Radial basis function neural network
ReLU	Rectified linear unit
RF	Radio frequency (Chap. 2)
RF	Random forest (Chaps. 8 and 11)
RKPCA	Radial basis function kernel principal component analysis
RN	Repetition number
ROI	Region of interest
RQ	Rayleigh quotient
RSA	Restarted simulated annealing
RST	Rough set theory
SA	Simulated annealing
SAE	Sparse autoencoder
SAH	Subarachnoid hemorrhage
SCGD	Scaled conjugate gradient descent
SCV	Stratified cross validation
SDE	Semidefinite embedding
SI	Swarm intelligence
SIV	Suitability index variable
SL	Supervised learning
SNP	Sliding neighborhood processing
SNR	Signal-to-noise ratio
SPAIR	Spectrally adiabatic inversion recovery
SPECT	Single-photon emission computed tomography
SPM	Statistical parametric mapping
SSL	Semi-supervised learning
STFT	Short-time Fourier transform
STIR	short T_1 inversion recovery

STT	Student's t-test
SVM	Support vector machine
SVS	Single-voxel spectroscopy
SWI	Susceptibility weighted imaging
SWT	Stationary wavelet transform
TE	Echo time
TIA	Transient ischemic attack
TL	Tabu list
TLE	Temporal lobe epilepsy
TR	Repetition time
TS	Tabu search
TSVM	Twin support vector machine
UTFD	Unified time–frequency domain
UWT	Undecimated wavelet transform
WM	White matter
WNN	Weighted nearest neighbor
WPT	Wavelet packet transform
WT	Wavelet transform
WTA	Winner-take-all
WTT	Welch's t-test
ZM	Zernike moment
ZP	Zernike polynomial

List of Figures

Chapter 1
Basics of Pathological Brain Detection

Pathological brain detection (PBD) systems help neuroradiologists to make assisted decisions based on brain images. At present, there are two types of PBD systems. Type I is aimed at detecting all types of brain disease, and its detection rate is improving gradually. Type II is aimed at detecting specific brain diseases, and then integrating all these in a system. Both types of system are hot research topics. This chapter first introduces the history of pathological brain detection. It then goes on to divide common brain diseases into four categories: neoplastic disease, neurodegeneration, cerebrovascular disease, and inflammation. We also give a standard computer-aided pathological brain detection prototype. Finally, promising research trends are predicted.

1.1 History

The development of PBD can be divided into three stages: from the 1990s, based on knowledge and experience obtained from neuroradiologists, computer scientists developed PBD using so-called "knowledge-based system" or "expert system" techniques. The employed features are commonly understandable to humans, such as cortical thickness, area of particular brain tissue, etc. Cavestri et al. [1] presented an expert system, "*Focus*," for locating acute neurological events. Brai et al. [2] developed the "EPEXS" for evoking potential analysis and interpretation. Juhola et al. [3] compared expert systems with human expertise, and proved, at an abstract level, that they complemented each other. Imran et al. [4] developed an expert system that detected cerebral blood flow (CBF) deficits in neuropsychiatric disorders.

Later, computer scientists realized that mathematical features (shape, texture, statistical, etc.) could also achieve equivalent or even better performance than features understandable to humans, therefore, scholars tended to add advanced image features, such as wavelets and gray-level co-occurrence matrices (GLCM).

© Springer Nature Singapore Pte Ltd. 2018
S.-H. Wang et al., *Pathological Brain Detection*, Brain Informatics and Health,
https://doi.org/10.1007/978-981-10-4026-9_1

Terae et al. [5] used a wavelet compression technique to detect brain lesions. Barra and Boire [6] used 3D wavelet representation for tissue segmentation. Antel et al. [7] employed GLCM to lateralize seizure focus in temporal lobe epilepsy (TLE) patients using normal volumetric magnetic resonance imaging (MRI).

Moreover, the successes of pattern recognition (PR) have been reported in breast cancer [8], edge detection [9], cancer diagnosis [10], aerial vehicle [11], electroencephalograms (EEGs) [12], review identification [13], etc. Such successes suggested that scholars should use PR techniques to detect pathological brains. PR systems with labeled training data are called "supervised learning (SL)" systems and those with no labeled data are called "unsupervised learning" systems. SL is commonly used in PBD, since it allows neuroradiologists to label the data.

Recently, various optimization techniques have been proposed and applied to train classifiers in order to increase detection performance. Traditional classifier training used gradient descent–based methods; nevertheless, the complicated optimization surfaces and discretized version of the problem meant that gradient-based methods suffered from falling into local best points. Hence, new meta-heuristic optimization methods have been proposed. Dorigo [14] proposed an ant colony optimization (ACO) algorithm based on an ant colony. Kennedy and Eberhart [15] proposed a particle swarm optimization (PSO) algorithm based on bird's flocking. Besides these, differential evolution (DE) [16], artificial bee colony optimization [17], glowworm swarm optimization (GSO) [18], and many other excellent optimization techniques have been proposed.

1.2 Brain Diseases

Many different types of brain disease exist. We can divide them, roughly, into four categories [19] as shown in Table 1.1.

Table 1.1 Four categories of brain disease

Category	Common diseases
Neoplastic disease	Glioma, metastatic bronchogenic carcinoma, meningioma, sarcoma, astrocytoma, oligodendroglioma, metastatic adenocarcinoma
Neurodegeneration	Parkinson's disease, Alzheimer's disease, Huntington's disease, motor neuron disease (amyotrophic lateral sclerosis), Pick's disease, cerebral calcinosis, Batten disease, prion disease, spinocerebellar ataxia, Friedreich's ataxia
Cerebrovascular disease	Cerebral hemorrhage, acute stroke, hypertensive encephalopathy, multiple embolic infarction, subacute stroke, vascular dementia, chronic subdural hematoma, cavernous angioma, subarachnoid hemorrhage, fatal stroke, transient ischemic attack
Inflammation	Encephalitis, cerebral toxoplasmosis, multiple sclerosis, abscess, Lyme encephalopathy, AIDS dementia, herpes encephalitis, Creutzfeldt–Jakob disease, meningitis, vasculitis

1.2.1   Neoplastic Disease

The first category we shall consider is neoplastic disease (also called tumors) [20]. Primary neoplastic disease starts in brain and remains there, while secondary neoplastic disease starts elsewhere and then travels to the brain. Benign tumors do not have cancer cells, rarely spread, and may cause problems if pressing against certain brain areas. Malignant tumors have cancer cells and invade healthy tissues nearby.

Four grades of brain tumors are listed in Table 1.2. A Grade I tumor is rare in adults and is associated with long-term survival. A Grade II tumor will sometimes spread into nearby tissues, and may come back as a higher grade tumor. Grade III and IV tumors actively reproduce abnormal cells. Grade IV is extremely dangerous: it forms new blood vessels to maintain rapid growth and contains necrosis in its center, as shown in Fig. 1.1. Effective treatments include surgery, radiation therapy, chemotherapy, and combined therapies [21].

1.2.2   Neurodegeneration

The second category of brain disease is neurodegeneration, viz., the progressive loss (even death) in structure or function of neurons [22]. Neurons normally do not reproduce, so they cannot be replaced after being damaged. Neurodegeneration diseases are incurable, and lead to progressive degeneration.

Figure 1.2 shows three tissues which can be used to distinguishing between Alzheimer's disease (AD) and a normal control. The first is the shrinkage seen in the cerebral cortex. The second is the enlargement of the ventricle. The third is the shrinkage seen in the hippocampus. Figure 1.3 shows the neurofibrillary tangles in AD patients.

Neurodegeneration affects many daily activities by affecting muscles, movement, balance, talking, heart function, sleep, etc. It also causes problems in mental functioning.

1.2.3   Cerebrovascular Disease

The third category of brain disease is cerebrovascular disease [23]. It is a severe medical condition, which is caused by affecting the blood supply to the brain. Four common cerebrovascular diseases are:

Table 1.2 Four grades of brain tumors

Grade	Growth speed	Appearance under a microscope
I	Slow	Almost normal
II	Relatively slow	Slightly abnormal
III	Relatively fast	Abnormal
IV	Fast	Very abnormal

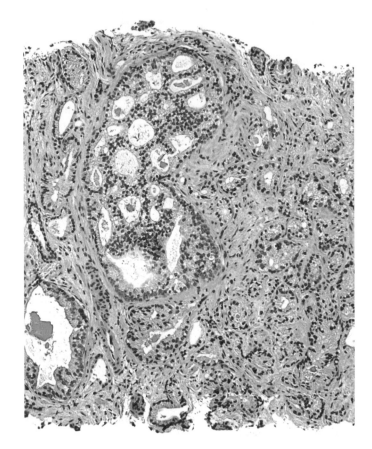

Fig. 1.1 Prostate cancer cell

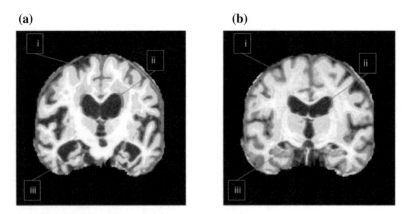

Fig. 1.2 a Brain affected by Alzheimer's disease. **b** A normal brain

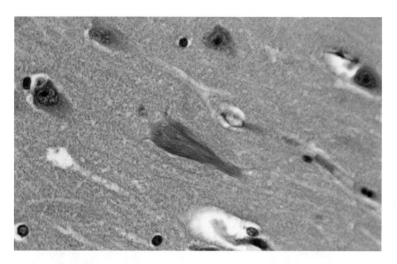

Fig. 1.3 The neurofibrillary tangles in Alzheimer's disease

1. A stroke, which happens when the blood supply is blocked or interrupted by a clot, causing parts of the brain to die due to cerebral infarction.
2. A transient ischemic attack (TIA) [24], which is caused by temporary blood disruption. It is also called a "mini-stroke" with symptoms resolving within 24 h.
3. A subarachnoid hemorrhage (SAH), which happens when blood leaks from arteries, located underneath the arachnoid, to the brain surface.
4. Vascular dementia, which is caused by brain cell damage due to a complex interaction of cerebrovascular diseases.

Figure 1.4 shows coarctation of the aorta. This disease can raise the likelihood of heart failure.

1.2.4   Inflammation

Finally, the fourth category is inflammatory disease [25]. We all know that the brain is protected by the calvarium, dura, and blood–brain barrier (BBB). The cerebral tissue is relatively resistant to invading infections. Nevertheless, the brain or the spinal cord can become inflamed, leading to swelling and irritation of tissues or vessels. Inflammatory diseases include abscess, meningitis, encephalitis, and vasculitis. Initially, inflammatory control is used to prevent inflammation-induced organ destruction. After that, medication is prescribed to control the symptoms. Finally, control of uncomfortable side effects is necessary, induced by many of the treatments.

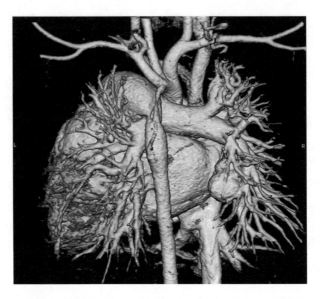

Fig. 1.4 The coarctation of the aorta may increase the likelihood of heart failure

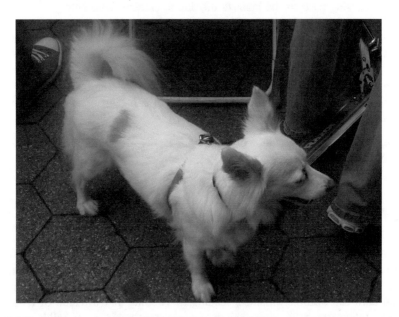

Fig. 1.5 Rabies can be passed from infected dogs through biting

Figure 1.5 shows a dog infected with rabies (also called hydrophobia). Viral inflammation of the human brain can be caused by dog bites to the muscles. Figure 1.6 shows a brain tissue biopsy of a patient with Creutzfeldt–Jakob disease (CJD).

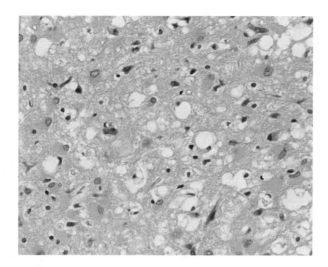

Fig. 1.6 Brain tissue biopsy from a patient with Creutzfeldt–Jakob disease

1.2.5   Summary

According to mortality rates reported in 2002, cardiovascular disease is responsible for 29.34% of deaths, which is more than any other disease (Table 1.3). Infectious diseases (including brain inflammation outlined in this chapter) ranks second and accounts for 23.04% of deaths. Neoplasm (including brain neoplastic disease outlined in this chapter) ranks third and accounts for 12.49% of deaths. This demonstrates the importance of this book.

1.3   A Standard Computer-Aided Diagnosis System

Figure 1.7 shows the block diagram for developing a computer-aided diagnosis (CAD) system for PBD using artificial intelligence (AI) in MRI. Roughly, we can divide the process into seven steps [26]:

Table 1.3 Mortality rates (released in 2012)

Rank	Cause	Causes of death (%)
1	Cardiovascular disease	29.34
2	Infectious disease	23.04
3	Neoplasm	12.49
4	Respiratory disease	6.49
5	Unintentional injury	6.23
6	Digestive disease	3.45
7	Intentional jury	2.84
8	Neuropsychiatric disorder	1.95

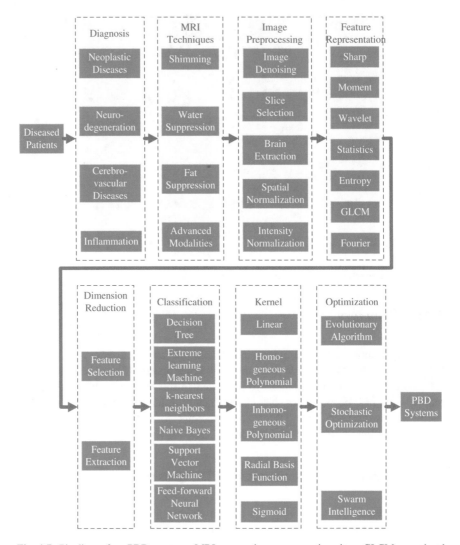

Fig. 1.7 Pipeline of a PBD system. MRI magnetic resonance imaging; GLCM gray-level co-occurrence matrix; pathological brain detection

- Diagnosis.
- Imaging techniques.
- Image preprocessing.
- Feature representation.
- Dimension reduction.
- Classification (kernel).
- Optimization methods.

In the text that follows, we will expatiate each block.

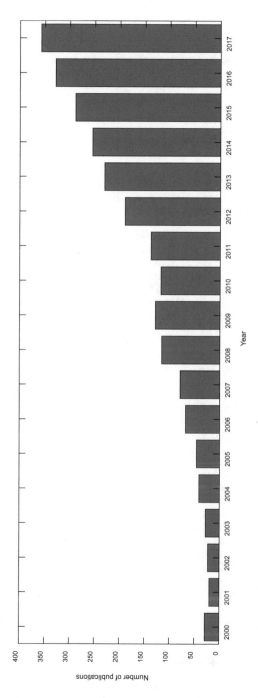

Fig. 1.8 Publication trend (data obtained on 1 April 2018)

1.4 Research Trends

Figure 1.8 shows the trend in related publications over the years. The results show that research on this topic is increasing steadily over time. Moreover, this picture also validates the topic of this book which receives intense attention from international scholars.

References

1. Cavestri R, Radice L, D'Angelo V, Longhini E (1991) Focus. An expert system for the clinical diagnosis of the location of acute neurologic events (Focus. Un sistema esperto per la diagnosi clinica di sede di incidenti neurologici a comparsa acuta). Minerva Med 82(12):815–820
2. Brai A, Vibert J-F, Koutlidis R (1994) An expert system for the analysis and interpretation of evoked potentials based on fuzzy classification: application to brainstem auditory evoked potentials. Comput Biomed Res 27(5):351–366. https://doi.org/10.1006/cbmr.1994.1027
3. Juhola M, Auramo Y, Kentala E, Pyykko I (1995) An essay on power of expert systems versus human expertise. Med Inf 20(2):133–138.
4. Imran MB, Kawashima R, Sato K, Kinomura S, Ono S, Qureshy A, Fukuda H (1999) Detection of CBF deficits in neuropsychiatric disorders by an expert system: a 99Tcm-HMPAO brain SPET study using automated image registration. Nucl Med Commun 20(1):25–32. https://doi.org/10.1097/00006231-199901000-00006
5. Terae S, Miyasaka K, Kudoh K, Nambu T, Yoshikawa H, Shimizu T, Fujita N (1998) Wavelet compression on detection of brain lesions at MR imaging in teleradiology. In: Lemke HU, Vannier MW, Inamura K, Farman AG (eds) International Congress Series, vol 1165. International Congress Series. Elsevier Science Publishers, pp 459–463
6. Barra V, Boire JY (2000) Tissue segmentation on MR images of the brain by possibilistic clustering on a 3D wavelet representation. JMRI–J Magn Reson Imaging 11(3):267–278. https://doi.org/10.1002/(sici)1522-2586(200003)
7. Antel SB, Bernasconi N, Andermann F, Bernasconi A (2003) Texture analysis lateralizes seizure focus in TLE patients with normal volumetric MRI. Epilepsia 44(Supplement 9):255
8. Fusco R, Sansone M, Filice S, Carone G, Amato DM, Sansone C, Petrillo A (2016) Pattern recognition approaches for breast cancer DCE-MRI classification: a systematic review. J Med Biol Eng 36(4):449–459. https://doi.org/10.1007/s40846-016-0163-7
9. James AP (2016) Edge detection for pattern recognition: a survey. Int J Appl Pattern Recogn 3(1):1–21. https://doi.org/10.1504/ijapr.2016.076980
10. Abarghouei AA, Ghanizadeh A, Sinaie S, Shamsuddin SM (2009) A survey of pattern recognition applications in cancer diagnosis. In: Abraham A, Muda AK, Herman NS, Shamsuddin SM, Huoy CY (eds), International conference of soft computing and pattern recognition, Malacca, Malaysia. IEEE, pp 448–453. https://doi.org/10.1109/socpar.2009.93
11. Raut O, Conrad JM, Willis AR (2011) Survey of recognition of Arabic scripts for indoor unmanned aerial vehicles using classical methods for pattern recognition. In: IEEE Southeastcon 2011: building global engineers, New York IEEE SoutheastCon-Proceedings. IEEE, pp 255–259
12. Bularka S, Gontean A (2015) EEG pattern recognition techniques review. In: 21st International symposium for design and technology in electronic packaging (SIITME), Brasov, Romania. IEEE, pp 273–276
13. van der Meer J, Frasincar F (2013) Automatic review identification on the web using pattern recognition. Softw-Pract Experience 43(12):1415–1436. https://doi.org/10.1002/spe.2152

14. Dorigo M (1992) Optimization, learning and natural algorithms. Politecnico di Milano, Italy
15. Kennedy J, Eberhart R (1995) Particle swarm optimization. In: IEEE international conference on neural networks. IEEE, pp 1942–1948. https://doi.org/10.1109/icnn.1995.488968
16. Storn R, Price K (1997) Differential evolution—a simple and efficient heuristic for global optimization over continuous spaces. J Global Optim 11(4):341–359. https://doi.org/10.1023/a:1008202821328
17. Karaboga D, Basturk B (2007) Artificial Bee Colony (ABC) optimization algorithm for solving constrained optimization problems. In: Melin P, Castillo O, Aguilar LT, Kacprzyk J, Pedrycz W (eds) Foundations of fuzzy logic and soft computing, vol 4529. Lecture notes in computer science. Springer-Verlag Press, Berlin, pp 789–798
18. Krishnanand KN, Ghose D (2005) Detection of multiple source locations using a glowworm metaphor with applications to collective robotics. In: IEEE swarm intelligence symposium, Pasadena. IEEE, pp 84–91. https://doi.org/10.1109/sis.2005.1501606
19. Zhan T (2016) Pathological brain detection by artificial intelligence in magnetic resonance imaging scanning. Prog Electromagnet Res 156:105–133
20. Paliogiannis P, Scognamillo F, Attene F, Marrosu A, Trignano E, Tedde L, Delogu D, Trignano M (2013) Preneoplastic and neoplastic gallbladder lesions occasionally discovered after elective video cholecystectomy for benign disease. A single centre experience and literature review. Ann Ital Chir 84(3):281–285
21. Martinez-Gonzalez A, Duran-Prado M, Calvo GF, Alcain FJ, Perez-Romasanta LA, Perez-Garcia VM (2015) Combined therapies of antithrombotics and antioxidants delay in silico brain tumour progression. Math Med Biol 32(3):239–262. https://doi.org/10.1093/imammb/dqu002
22. Vasapolli R, Schulz C, Ner DB, Heinze H, Malfertheiner P (2016) New insights into the roles of gut microbiota in neurodegenerative diseases: a systematic review. Helicobacter 21:171–171
23. Smeeing DPJ, Hendrikse J, Petersen ET, Donahue MJ, de Vis JB (2016) Arterial spin labeling and blood oxygen level-dependent MRI cerebrovascular reactivity in cerebrovascular disease: a systematic review and meta-analysis. Cerebrovasc Dis 42(3–4):288–307. https://doi.org/10.1159/000446081
24. Oostema JA, Brown MD, Reeves M (2016) Emergency department management of transient ischemic attack: a survey of emergency physicians. J Stroke Cerebrovasc Dis 25(6):1517–1523. https://doi.org/10.1016/j.jstrokecerebrovasdis.2016.02.028
25. Byrne ML, Whittle S, Allen NB (2016) The role of brain structure and function in the association between inflammation and depressive symptoms: a systematic review. Psychosom Med 78(4):389–400. https://doi.org/10.1097/psy.0000000000000311
26. Phillips P, Dong Z, Yang J (2015) Pathological brain detection in magnetic resonance imaging scanning by wavelet entropy and hybridization of biogeography-based optimization and particle swarm optimization. Prog Electromagnet Res 152:41–58. https://doi.org/10.2528/PIER15040602

Chapter 2
Neuroimaging Modalities

This chapter briefly introduces the development of neuroimaging modalities. We give a simple introduction about pneumoencephalography (PEG), cerebral angiography, computerized tomography, and nuclear imaging (positron emission tomography and single photon emission computed tomography). Later in the chapter, the technique of magnetic resonance imaging (MRI) is considered. Projectile risk, shimming technique, and water and fat suppression are discussed, with two contrasting types (spin–lattice and spin–spin) of MRI. A method for rough interpretation of magnetic resonance images is given. Finally, we make a comparison among different imaging modalities in MRI, including diffusion tensor imaging, functional MRI, magnetic resonance angiography, and magnetic resonance spectral imaging.

2.1 History of Neuroimaging

Neuroimaging uses various techniques to show the structure or function of the brain [1, 2]. It is interdisciplinary, combining medicine, neuroscience, psychology, computer science, etc. Two categories comprise neuroimaging:

- Structural imaging.
- Functional imaging.

2.1.1 Pneumoencephalography

Ventriculography was a primitive method where air was injected through holes drilled in the skull. In 1918, the technique of "pneumoencephalography" was proposed by Walter Dandy. This technique drains the cerebrospinal fluid

© Springer Nature Singapore Pte Ltd. 2018
S.-H. Wang et al., *Pathological Brain Detection*, Brain Informatics and Health,
https://doi.org/10.1007/978-981-10-4026-9_2

(CSF) using a lumbar puncture [3], and then replaces the CSF with a mixture of oxygen, air, and helium, to allow the brain structure to show clearly on an X-ray imaging scan [4]. Figure 2.1 shows an image obtained using PEG.

2.1.2 Cerebral Angiography

In 1927, a Portuguese neurologist, Egas Moniz, developed the cerebral angiography. For this technique a catheter is inserted into a large artery and a contrast agent injected [5]. Imaging is implemented when the contrast agent spreads through the arterial and the venous system within the brain [6]. Figure 2.2 shows an image obtained using cerebral angiography.

Fig. 2.1 An image obtained using PEG

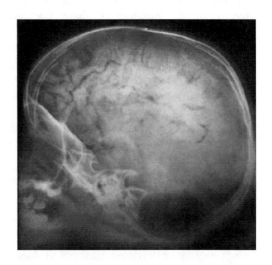

Fig. 2.2 An image obtained using cerebral angiography

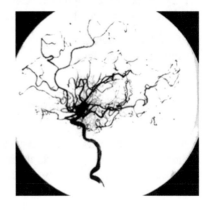

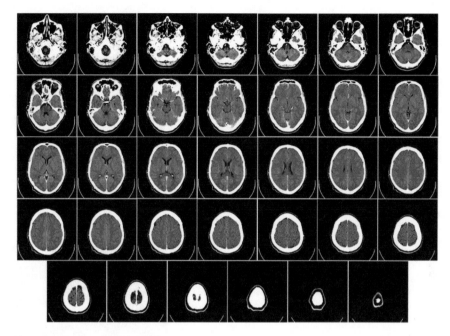

Fig. 2.3 CT images of the human brain

2.1.3 Computerized Tomography

In 1970, Godfrey Newbold Hounsfield and Allan M. Cormack developed computerized tomography (CT). This technique provides images of the detailed anatomic structure within the brain, as shown in Fig. 2.3. In 1979, they shared the Nobel Prize in Physiology or Medicine.

2.1.4 Positron Emission Tomography

Later, using radioligands, positron emission tomography (PET) and single-photon emission computed tomography (SPECT) were carried out within the brain.

PET observes metabolic processers [7]. It is used in both clinical oncology and diagnosis. PET is also heavily used in pre-clinical studies on animals for cancer research.

For example, if the biologically active molecule used is fludeoxyglucose (FDG) [8], the image will indicate tissue metabolic activity corresponding to regional glucose uptake. Figure 2.4 shows an example of a brain PET image. Figure 2.5 shows an example of a kidney PET image.

Fig. 2.4 PET image of the brain

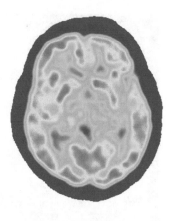

Fig. 2.5 PET image of a kidney

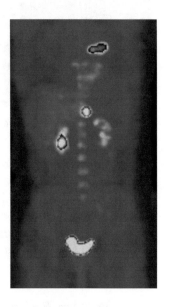

2.1.5   Single-Photon Emission Computed Tomography

SPECT is another important nuclear imaging technique using gamma rays. It is able to provide true 3D information. It injects a radionuclide into the brain's bloodstream [9]. Usually, a marker radioisotope is linked to a specific ligand to form the radioligand. Ligand concentration is detected by a gamma camera.

Table 2.1 presents six common SPECT protocols for different studies. For the brain, technetium-99m is usually used [10] —being a radioisotope with an emission energy of 140 keV. Figure 2.6 shows a SPECT image of the brain.

Table 2.1 Common SPECT protocols

Study	Radioisotope	Emission energy (keV)
Bone	Technetium-99m	140
Myocardial perfusion	Technetium-99m	140
Sestamibi parathyroid	Technetium-99m	140
Brain	Technetium-99m	140
Neuroendocrine	Iodine-123 or iodine-131	159
White cells	Indium-111	171

Fig. 2.6 SPECT image of the brain

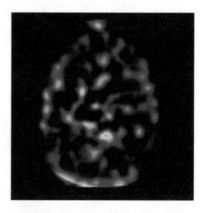

2.2 Magnetic Resonance Imaging

Paul Lauterbur and Peter Mansfield concurrently designed the MRI technique. They shared the Nobel Prize in Physiology or Medicine in 2003. The technique uses both magnetic fields and pulses in order to generate pictures of brain's anatomy [11]. Different tissues provide direct contrasts, due to the different relaxation properties of the hydrogen atoms they contain. MRI is radiation free [12, 13]. Figure 2.7 shows a Siemens MR scanner.

2.2.1 Projectile Risk

MRI is safe and painless. It does not involve radiation [14]. Nevertheless, Fig. 2.8 shows that patients with heart pacemakers, cochlear implants, metal dentures, and metal implants cannot be scanned, because of the extremely high-strength magnets used. This is called the projectile (or missile) effect and is shown in Fig. 2.9. It refers to the dangerous ability of an MRI scanner to attract ferromagnetic, iron-based materials.

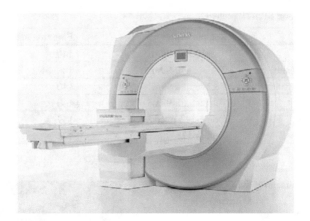

Fig. 2.7 A Siemens MR scanner

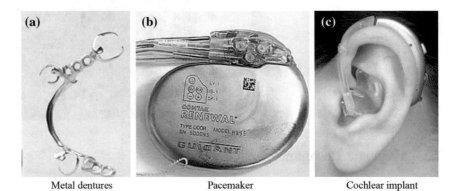

Metal dentures   Pacemaker   Cochlear implant

Fig. 2.8 Examples of metal gadgets which should be removed before scanning

Fig. 2.9 A wheel chair
which crashed into an MRI
scanner in Shanghai

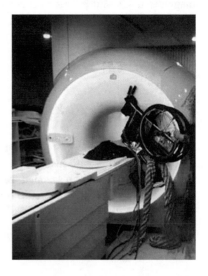

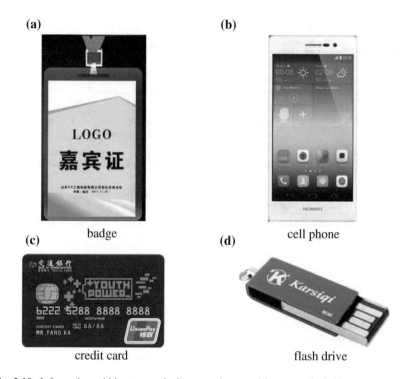

(a)

badge

(b)

cell phone

(c)

credit card

(d)

flash drive

Fig. 2.10 Information within storage devices may be erased by magnetic fields

Such a powerful magnet can also erase information from storage devices, such as ID badges, cell phones, subway cards, credit cards, flash drives, etc. Figure 2.10 shows four such devices affected by magnetic fields.

2.2.2 Shimming

Shimming is undertaken to correct the inhomogeneity of the magnetic field produced by the main magnet in the scanner. The inhomogeneity may arise from both imperfections in the magnet and the presence of external objects (such as the brain).

In active shimming, currents are directed through dedicated coils in order to improve homogeneity. In passive shimming, small pieces of sheet metal are inserted within the scanner bore [15].

Active shimming coils can be either superconducting or resistive. Both active and passive shimming are controlled by specialized circuitry, needing its own power supply [16].

Table 2.2 Comparison of fat suppression techniques

Technique	Advantage	Disadvantage
STIR	Insensitive to B_0 inhomogeneity	Increased minimal TR and total measurement time; tissue contrast affected
Dixon	Insensitive to B_0 and B_1 inhomogeneity	Minimal TR increased
Water selective excitation	Insensitive to B_1 inhomogeneity	Increased minimum TE, TR, and total measurement time
Spectral fat saturation	Shorter TR; tissue contrast preserved	Sensitive to B_0 and B_1 inhomogeneity
SPAIR	Insensitive to B_1 inhomogeneity; tissue contrast preserved	Increased minimal TR

Notes B_0, a constant and homogeneous magnetic field to polarize spins; B_1, an RF magnetic field perpendicular to B_0; TE, echo time; TR, repetition time

2.2.3 Water and Fat Suppression

Hydrogen atoms can generate a detectable radio frequency (RF) signal, and they are abundant in both water and fat in the human body. To balance image contrast, water suppression and fat suppression are necessary in some particular MRI scans.

Water suppression can be implemented by presaturation [17], flip-back [18], and "jump and return" [19].

Fat suppression is based on the fact that hydrogen nuclei in fat tissues have different values for MRI-related parameters [20]. Two types of fat suppression techniques exist:

1. Relaxation-dependent techniques, such as short T_1 inversion recovery (STIR).
2. Chemical shift–dependent techniques, including Dixon, water selective excitation [21], spectral fat saturation [22], and spectrally adiabatic inversion recovery (SPAIR) [23].

A comparison of these fat suppression methods is given in Table 2.2.

2.2.4 Two Types of Contrast

Different image contrast can emphasize different anatomical structures. There are two common types of image contrasts: T_1 (also known as spin–lattice) relaxation [24] and T_2 (also known as spin–spin) relaxation [25].

T_1 characterizes the rate at which the longitudinal component M_z of the magnetization vector recovers exponentially toward its equilibrium M_{eq}. Mathematically given as:

$$M_z(t) = M_{eq}\left(1 - e^{-t/T_1}\right) \tag{2.1}$$

T_2 characterizes the time for the magnetic resonance signal M_{xy} to decay to about 37% (1/e) of its initial value, after its generation by tipping the longitudinal magnetization toward the transverse plane:

$$M_{xy}(t) = M_{xy}(0) \times e^{-t/T_2} \tag{2.2}$$

Figure 2.11 shows the relaxation curves of T_1 and T_2. Figure 2.12 shows two images, using both contrast types, of the same slice. In general, the T_1 image is suitable to assess the cerebral cortex, and the T_2 image is suitable to assess inflammation and white matter lesions [26].

2.2.5 Interpretation

The interpretation of T_1 and T_2 MR images are given in Tables 2.3 and 2.4. Roughly, the brain segmentation represents a three-class classification problem: gray matter (GM), white matter (WM), and cerebrospinal fluid (CSF). The comparison of GM and WM are listed in the intermediate gray-levels.

The pathological process increases water content in neighboring tissues. The additional water decreases the signal in T_1 image, and meanwhile increases the signal in the T_2 image [27]. Therefore, pathological processes are more visible in the T_2 image than in the T_1 image [28].

2.3 Other Magnetic Resonance Imaging Modalities

2.3.1 Diffusion Tensor Imaging

Diffusion tensor imaging (DTI) measures the diffusion of water molecules within the brain, so as to produce neural tract images [29].

Each voxel in DTI is calculated from a vector or matrix from more than six different diffusion weighted acquisitions (Fig. 2.13a). The fiber directions are calculated from DTI data using particular algorithms (Fig. 2.13b).

2.3.2 Functional Magnetic Resonance Imaging

Functional magnetic resonance imaging (fMRI) is used to measure brain activity—responses to external stimuli or passive activity in a resting state [30]. It is based on

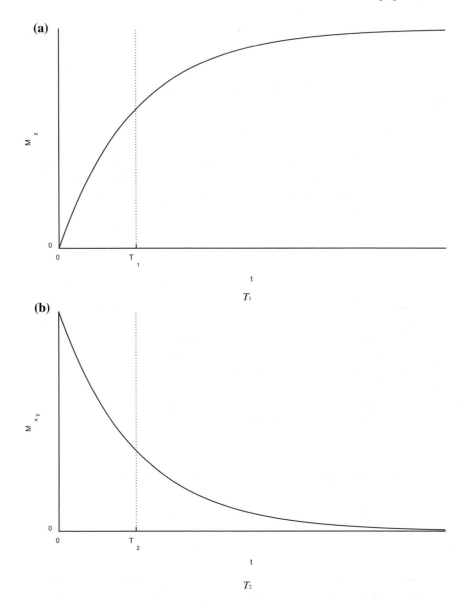

Fig. 2.11 Relaxation curves

the blood oxygen level–dependent (BOLD) contrast, by imaging the changes in blood flow related to energy used by cells in the brain [31]. Figure 2.14 presents two images of an fMRI scan with activation regions in a pseudo-colormap.

(a)   **(b)**

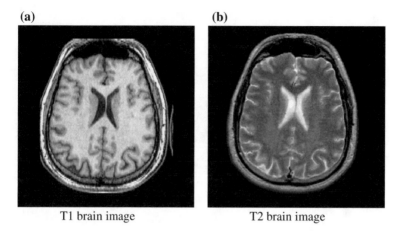

T1 brain image   T2 brain image

Fig. 2.12 Two contrast images of the same brain slice

Table 2.3 Interpretation of T_1-weighted image

Gray-level	Tissue
Bright	Fat
Intermediate	GM is darker than WM
Dark	Bone, air, water

Table 2.4 Interpretation of T_2-weighted image

Gray-level	Tissue
Bright	Water
Intermediate	WM is darker than GM
Dark	Bone, air, fat

2.3.3   Magnetic Resonance Angiography

Magnetic resonance angiography (MRA) aims at imaging blood vessels [32]. It generates images of arteries and veins to evaluate for stenosis, occlusions, aneurysms, and other abnormalities in vessels [33]. To display 3D angiography, computers use the maximum intensity project (MIP) technique to simulate rays through the volume, selecting the highest value to display on screen (Figure 2.15).

2.3.4   Magnetic Resonance Spectroscopic Imaging

Magnetic resonance spectroscopic imaging (MRSI) measures the levels of different metabolites (Fig. 2.16) in any position within the brain. Two simpler techniques are single-voxel spectroscopy (SVS) and chemical shift imaging (CSI).

(a)   **(b)**

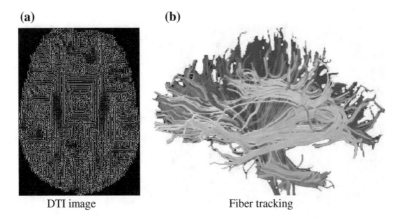

DTI image   Fiber tracking

Fig. 2.13   Illustration of a DTI image and tracked fibers

Fig. 2.14   An fMRI image
showing activation regions

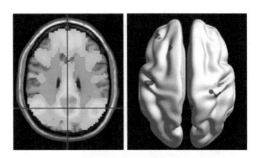

Fig. 2.15   An illustration of
an MRA image

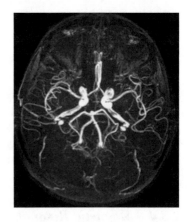

Clinically, MRSI can detect metabolic changes associated with strokes, autism, brain tumors, multiple sclerosis, seizures, depression, Parkinson's disease, Kimura disease, etc. It can also be used in animal medicine. Table 2.5 lists MRSI identifiable metabolites (N-acetyl aspartate, choline, creatine, lipid, lactate, myo-inositol,

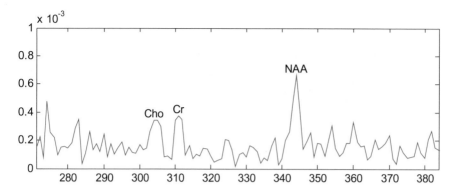

Fig. 2.16 An example of MRSI

Table 2.5 Metabolities in MRSI

Metabolite	Position	Indications
N-acetyl aspartate	Major peak at 2.02 ppm	Its decrease suggests loss or damage to neuronal tissue
Choline	Major peak at 3.2 ppm	Its increase suggests an increase in membrane breakdown or cell production
Creatine	Major peak at 3.0 ppm	Its decrease may suggest tissue death or major cell death. Its increase could be from craniocerebral trauma
Lipid	Major aliphatic peaks in 0.9–1.5 ppm	Its increase suggests necrosis
Lactate	A doublet at 1.33 ppm	Its presence suggests glycolysis in an oxygen-deficient environment, which may arise from ischemia, hypoxia, mitochondrial disorders, and tumors
Myo-inositol	Major peak at 3.56 ppm	Its increase suggests AD, dementia, and HIV
Glutamate and glutamine	Resonance peaks at 2.2–2.4 ppm	Its increase may suggest hyperammonemia or hepatic encephalopathy

Notes AD Alzheimer's disease; HIV human immunodeficiency virus

glutamate and glutamine), and gives their peak positions and indications of change. The peaks are measured in parts per million (ppm). Note that the lipid spectrum is easily contaminated, because of fat located in the scalp and underneath the skull.

2.4 Conclusion

In this chapter, popular neuroimaging modalities have been discussed. Their strengths and weaknesses have been revealed and compared. New and powerful neuroimaging techniques are expected to emerge in the near future, which can help with exploration of the brain and central neural system.

References

1. Chakrabarty T, Ogrodniczuk J, Hadjipavlou G (2016) Predictive neuroimaging markers of psychotherapy response: a systematic review. Harvard Rev Psychiatry 24(6):396–405
2. Pidgeon LM, Grealy M, Duffy AHB, Hay L, McTeague C, Vuletic T, Coyle D, Gilbert SJ (2016) Functional neuroimaging of visual creativity: a systematic review and meta-analysis. Brain Behav 6(10), Article ID: e00540. https://doi.org/10.1002/brb3.540
3. Dumont CR, Guadalajara J, Varela S, Lupi E (1975) Myocardial infarct following left ventriculography. Report of 2 cases and review of the literature (Infarto del miocardio despues de una ventriculografia izquierda. Presentacion de dos casos y revision de la literatura). Arch Inst Cardiol Mex 45(2):178–187
4. Berger PB (1997) Diagnostic coronary angiography and ventriculography. Mayo Clinic cardiology review. Futura Publishing Co., Inc. Au: is this a book or journal—provide additional information please, that is publisher location or journal information. This is the book information: Berger PB (1997) Diagnostic coronary angiography and ventriculography. In: Murphy JG (ed) Mayo Clinic cardiology review. Futura Publishing Co., Inc., 135 Bedford Road, Armonk, New York 10504-0418, USA, pp 307–318. ISBN: 0-87993-662-2
5. Foss-Skiftesvik J, Snoer AH, Wagner A, Hauerberg J (2014) Transient global amnesia after cerebral angiography still occurs: case report and literature review. Radiol Case Rep 9(4):988. https://doi.org/10.2484/rcr.v9i4.988
6. Barata Tavares J, Leite I, Rodrigues D, Reimao S, Leitao J, Sequeira P (2012) Double aortic arch: incidental cerebral angiography finding in an adult patient with headache—embrionary cardiovascular morphogenic pattern review. Acta Med Port 25:45–47
7. Lopci E, Chiti A, Lazzeri M (2016) New clinical indications for F-18/C-11-choline, new tracers for positron emission tomography and a promising hybrid device for prostate cancer staging: a systematic review of the literature. Eur Urol 70(4):E112–E113. https://doi.org/10.1016/j.eururo.2016.03.025
8. Taghipour M, Sheikhbahaei S, Marashdeh W, Solnes L, Kiess A, Subramaniam RM (2016) Use of F-18-Fludeoxyglucose-Positron emission tomography/computed tomography for patient management and outcome in oropharyngeal squamous cell carcinoma. JAMA Otolaryngol-Head Neck Surg 142(1):79–85. https://doi.org/10.1001/jamaoto.2015.2607
9. Hess S, Frary EC, Gerke O, Madsen PH (2016) State-of-the-art imaging in pulmonary embolism: ventilation/perfusion single-photon emission computed tomography versus computed tomography angiography—controversies, results, and recommendations from a systematic review. Semin Thromb Hemost 42(8):833–845
10. Akbar MU, Ahmad MR, Shaheen A, Mushtaq S (2016) A review on evaluation of technetium-99m labeled radiopharmaceuticals. J Radioanal Nucl Chem 310(2):477–493. https://doi.org/10.1007/s10967-016-5019-7
11. De Vis JB, Alderliesten T, Hendrikse J, Petersen ET, Benders M (2016) Magnetic resonance imaging based noninvasive measurements of brain hemodynamics in neonates: a review. Pediatr Res 80(5):641–650. https://doi.org/10.1038/pr.2016.146

12. Dong Z, Phillips P, Ji G, Yang J (2015) Exponential wavelet iterative shrinkage thresholding algorithm for compressed sensing magnetic resonance imaging. Inf Sci 322:115–132. https://doi.org/10.1016/j.ins.2015.06.017

13. Phillips P, Dong Z, Ji G, Yang J (2015) Detection of Alzheimer's disease and mild cognitive impairment based on structural volumetric MR images using 3D-DWT and WTA-KSVM trained by PSOTVAC. Biomed Signal Process Control 21:58–73. https://doi.org/10.1016/j.bspc.2015.05.014

14. Yiu KCY, Greenspoon JN (2016) Clinical surveillance compared with clinical and magnetic resonance imaging surveillance for brain metastasis: a feasibility survey. Curr Oncol 23 (5):356–359. https://doi.org/10.3747/co.23.3155

15. Schmidt R, Webb A (2016) Improvements in RF shimming in high field MRI using high permittivity materials with low order pre-fractal geometries. IEEE Trans Med Imaging 35 (8):1837–1844. https://doi.org/10.1109/tmi.2016.2531120

16. Abe T (2016) B-1 homogeneity of breast MRI using RF shimming with individual specific values in volunteers simulating patients after mastectomy. Acta Radiol 57(11):1289–1296. https://doi.org/10.1177/0284185115585616

17. Goez M, Mok KH, Hore PJ (2005) Photo-CIDNP experiments with an optimized presaturation pulse train, gated continuous illumination, and a background-nulling pulse grid. J Magn Reson 177(2):236–246. https://doi.org/10.1016/j.jmr.2005.06.015

18. Lippens G, Dhalluin C, Wieruszeski JM (1995) Use of a water flip-back pulse in the homonuclear NOESY experiment. J Biomol NMR 5(3):327–331

19. Louis-Joseph A, Abergel D, Lebars I, Lallemand JY (2001) Enhancement of water suppression by radiation damping-based manipulation of residual water in Jump and Return NMR experiments. Chem Phys Lett 337(1–3):92–96. https://doi.org/10.1016/s0009-2614(01)00174-9

20. Takemori D, Kimura D, Yamada E, Higashida M (2016) Evaluation of fat suppression of diffusion-weighted imaging using section select gradient reversal technique on 3 T breast MRI. Nihon Hoshasen Gijutsu Gakkai Zasshi 72(7):589–594. https://doi.org/10.6009/jjrt.2016_JSRT_72.7.589

21. Deligianni X, Bar P, Scheffler K, Trattnig S, Bieri O (2014) Water-selective excitation of short T-2 species with binomial pulses. Magn Reson Med 72(3):800–805. https://doi.org/10.1002/mrm.24978

22. Clauser P, Pinker K, Helbich TH, Kapetas P, Bernathova M, Baltzer PAT (2014) Fat saturation in dynamic breast MRI at 3 Tesla: is the Dixon technique superior to spectral fat saturation? A visual grading characteristics study. Eur Radiol 24(9):2213–2219. https://doi.org/10.1007/s00330-014-3189-7

23. Choi WH, Oh SH, Lee CJ, Rhim JK, Chung BS, Hong HJ (2012) Usefulness of SPAIR image, fracture line and the adjacent discs change on magnetic resonance image in the acute osteoporotic compression fracture. Korean J Spine 9(3):227–231. https://doi.org/10.14245/kjs.2012.9.3.227

24. Yee S, Gao JH (2014) Effects of spin-lock field direction on the quantitative measurement of spin-lattice relaxation time constant in the rotating frame (T1 rho) in a clinical MRI system. Med Phys 41(12), Article ID: 122301. https://doi.org/10.1118/1.4900607

25. Yilmaz A, Yurdakoc M, Bernarding J, Vieth HM, Braun J, Yurt A (2002) Paramagnetic contribution of serum iron to the spin-spin relaxation rate (1/T-2) measured by MRI. Appl Magn Reson 22(1):11–22. https://doi.org/10.1007/bf03170519

26. Gullbrand SE, Ashinsky BG, Martin JT, Pickup S, Smith LJ, Mauck RL, Smith HE (2016) Correlations between quantitative T2 and T1 rho MRI, mechanical properties and biochemical composition in a rabbit lumbar intervertebral disc degeneration model. J Orthop Res 34 (8):1382–1388. https://doi.org/10.1002/jor.23269 Official Publication of the Orthopaedic Research Society

27. Bidhult S, Kantasis G, Aletras AH, Arheden H, Heiberg E, Hedstrom E (2016) Validation of T1 and T2 algorithms for quantitative MRI: performance by a vendor-independent software. BMC Med Imaging, 16, Article ID: 46. https://doi.org/10.1186/s12880-016-0148-6

28. Vairapperumal T, Saraswathy A, Ramapurath JS, Janardhanan SK, Unni NB (2016) Catechin tuned magnetism of Gd-doped orthovanadate through morphology as T-1-T-2 MRI contrast agents. Sci Rep 6, Article ID: 34976. https://doi.org/10.1038/srep34976

29. Kumar P, Yadav AK, Misra S, Kumar A, Chakravarty K, Prasad K (2016) Prediction of upper extremity motor recovery after subacute intracerebral hemorrhage through diffusion tensor imaging: a systematic review and meta-analysis. Neuroradiology 58(10):1043–1050. https://doi.org/10.1007/s00234-016-1718-6

30. Gaudio S, Wiemerslage L, Brooks SJ, Schioth HB (2016) A systematic review of resting-state functional-MRI studies in anorexia nervosa: Evidence for functional connectivity impairment in cognitive control and visuospatial and body-signal integration. Neurosci Biobehav Rev 71:578–589. https://doi.org/10.1016/j.neubiorev.2016.09.032

31. Weerakoon BS, Osuga T (2016) Characterization of flow distribution in the blood compartment of hollow fiber hemodialyzers with contrast-enhanced spin echo magnetic resonance imaging. Appl Magn Reson 47(4):453–469. https://doi.org/10.1007/s00723-016-0766-8

32. Di Leo G, Fisci E, Secchi F, Ali M, Ambrogi F, Sconfienza LM, Sardanelli F (2016) Diagnostic accuracy of magnetic resonance angiography for detection of coronary artery disease: a systematic review and meta-analysis. Eur Radiol 26(10):3706–3718. https://doi.org/10.1007/s00330-015-4134-0

33. Knuttinen M-G, Karow J, Mar W, Golden M, Xie KL (2014) Blood pool contrast-enhanced magnetic resonance angiography with correlation to digital subtraction angiography: a pictorial review. J Clin Imaging Sci 4:63. https://doi.org/10.4103/2156-7514.145860

Chapter 3
Image Preprocessing for Pathological Brain Detection

Image preprocessing is quite important. This chapter first introduces the concept of *k*-space, where the acquired signal lies. First, reconstruction is necessary to transform it to spatial space. Then, image denoising techniques are required. Magnetic resonance images are contaminated by Rician noise in addition to common Gaussian noise. Several denoising methods are introduced here. A brain extraction tool is introduced to strip the skull and preserve only brain tissues. The inter-class variance–based slice selection method is discussed, which aims to select one/several distinguishing slice(s). Spatial normalization is necessary, as it can transform a brain image to match a template. Rigid and non-rigid normalization methods are introduced. The intensity of normalization can improve image compatibility and facilitate comparability of scans with different settings. Finally, image enhancement is introduced, which can help improve the visual quality of magnetic brain images. Histogram equalization and contrast-limited adaptive histogram equalization methods are presented.

3.1 *k*-Space

Magnetic resonance (MR) scanners acquire signals and store them in *k*-space [1]. In practice, *k*-space refers to a temporary image space. When the *k*-space is full, the image reconstruction algorithm produces an image from the *k*-space to the image domain [2].

Selection of the spatial encoding involves the use of magnetic field gradients. Suppose the two directions in *k*-space are frequency encoding (FE) [3] and phase encoding (PE) [4, 5]; we can draw three examples of *k*-space of simulated phantom images below, in the first column in Fig. 3.1. The reconstructed images are shown in the last column in Fig. 3.1. These two representations may be converted from one to the other using the Fourier transform (FT) [6].

© Springer Nature Singapore Pte Ltd. 2018
S.-H. Wang et al., *Pathological Brain Detection*, Brain Informatics and Health,
https://doi.org/10.1007/978-981-10-4026-9_3

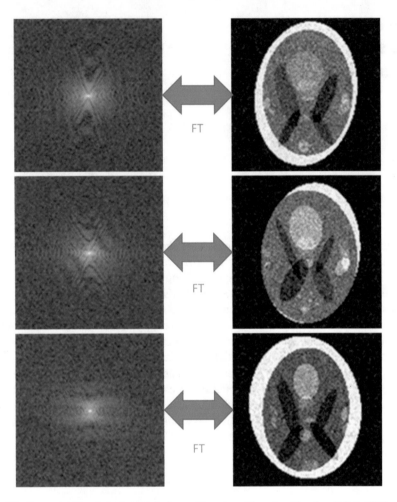

Fig. 3.1 Reconstruction from *k*-space (enhanced by a logarithm algorithm for clarity). *FT* Fourier transform

3.2 Image Denoising

3.2.1 Rician Noise

Image denoising is performed after image reconstruction. The random noise field in a low signal-to-noise ratio (SNR) MR image is described as Rician noise rather than Gaussian noise:

$$P(S, \sigma) = \frac{S}{\sigma^2} \exp\left(-\frac{S^2 + S_0^2}{2\sigma^2}\right) I_0\left(\frac{SS_0}{\sigma^2}\right) \tag{3.1}$$

where σ represents the standard deviation; S_0 is the true signal; S is the noise signal; and I_0 is the zeroth-order modified Bessel function [7].

3.2.2   Solutions

Some advanced image denoising methods were proposed to remove Rician noise. Figure 3.2 provides a visual example of denoising. Denoising algorithms should be edge preserving and must not blur important lesion information.

Iftikhar et al. [8] used an enhanced non-local means (NLM) algorithm. Phophalia et al. [9] explored the image space for each patch using rough set theory (RST). Yang et al. [10] proposed a pre-smoothing NLM filter. Phophalia and Mitra [11] used an RST-based bilateral filter (BF) to denoise brain images. Akar [12] also used a BF to eliminate noise. The parameters of a BF are optimized by a genetic algorithm (GA).

3.2.3   Wiener Filter

The Winner filter can alleviate Rician noise to some degree. The Matlab command "wiener2" uses a pixelwise adaptive Wiener method based on an estimation from the neighborhood of each pixel. Table 3.1 presents the details of this command.

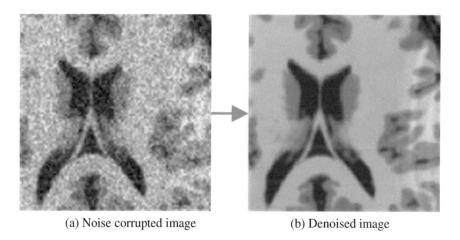

(a) Noise corrupted image   (b) Denoised image

Fig. 3.2   Rician noise removal

Table 3.1 The "wiener2" command

J = wiener2(I, [m n], np)
Input
I: Input image
[m n]: The size of neighborhood
np: noise power
Output
J: Denoised image

3.2.4 Wavelet-Based Denoising

Wavelets can also help with denoising. In this chapter, we will not expatiate wavelets, which will be introduced in Sect. 5.1. Three basic Matlab commands are introduced below:

- Command "wden" uses wavelets to denoise (Table 3.2).
- Command "wpdencmp" uses wavelet packets to denoise (Table 3.3).
- Command "wmulden" uses wavelets for multivariate denoising (Table 3.4).

Table 3.2 The "wden" command

XD = wden(X, TPTR, sh, SCAL, N, wname)
Input
X: Input image
TPTR: threshold selection rule (Stein's Unbiased risk, or its heuristic variant, or the universal threshold, or the minimax thresholding)
sh: soft or hard thresholding
SCAL: the multiplicative threshold rescaling
N: decomposition level
wname: wavelet name
Output
XD: denoised image

Table 3.3 The "wpdencmp" command

XD = wpdencmp(X, sh, N, wname, CRIT, PAR, ka)
Input
X: Input image
sh: soft or hard thresholding
N: decomposition level
wname: wavelet name
CRIT: criterion
PAR: parameter
ka[a]: keep approximation
Output
XD: denoised image
([a]If ka = 1, the approximation coefficients cannot be thresholded; if ka = 0, they can)

Table 3.4 The "wmulden" command

Y = wmulden(X, L, wname, npc_app, npc_fin, TPTR, sh)
Input
X: Input image
L: decomposition level
wname: wavelet name
npc_app: define the way to select principal components for approximation at level L in the wavelet domain
npc_fin: define the way to select principal components for final PCA after wavelet reconstruction
TPTR: threshold selection rule
sh: soft or hard thresholding
Output
Y: denoised image

3.3 Skull Stripping

It is necessary to remove the extra non-brain tissues (such as fat, skin, muscle, tissues in the neck, tongue, aponeurosis, meninges, periosteum, pharynx, eyeballs, etc.) from an MR image of the whole head, since they represent obstacles to automatic analysis [13]. This technique is called skull stripping. Non-brain tissues may decrease the performance of detecting brain diseases.

3.3.1 Software Library at the Oxford Centre for Functional MRI of the Brain

Skull-stripping methods were developed to solve this problem. Smith [14] presented a brain extraction tool (BET) in the software library (FSL) of the Oxford Centre for Functional MRI of the Brain (FMRIB). This tool is the most popular means of performing skull stripping.

The FSL is a comprehensive library created by the Analysis Group, FMRIB, Oxford, U.K. It can handle magnetic resonance imaging (MRI), diffusion tensor imaging (DTI), and functional magnetic resonance imaging (fMRI) formats efficiently and rapidly. The FSL can be installed in Mac OS X and Linux. For the Windows operating system, users need to install a virtual machine as shown in Fig. 3.3. Its main menu can be seen in Fig. 3.4.

Figures 3.5, 3.6, and 3.7 show BET results, highlighted in red, for sagittal, coronal, and axial views, respectively.

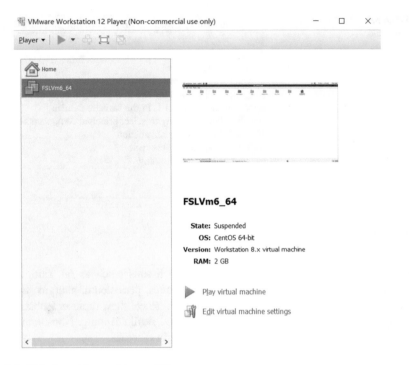

Fig. 3.3 Virtual machine used to run FSL

Fig. 3.4 The main menu of
the FSL

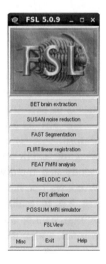

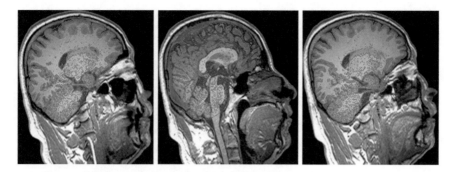

Fig. 3.5   Sagittal view of the brain extraction result using BET

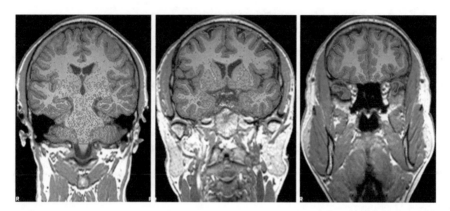

Fig. 3.6   Coronal view of the brain extraction result using BET

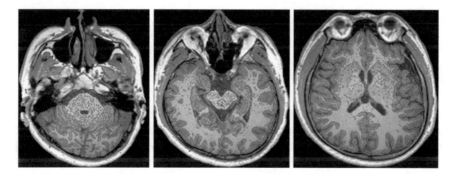

Fig. 3.7   Axial view of the brain extraction result using BET

Fig. 3.8 Start menu of SPM
(screenshot from the laptop of
the authors of this book)

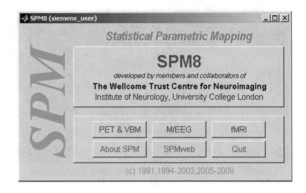

3.3.2   Statistical Parametric Mapping

Statistical parametric mapping (SPM) software is a toolbox working on Matlab. The
latest version is SPM12. Figure 3.8 presents its start menu.

SPM can also carry out skull stripping by segmenting a scanned image. It uses a
thresholded version of the sum of gray matter (GM) and white matter
(WM) probability maps to mask out the "bias-corrected structural scan."

Suppose the GM probability map is I_1, the WM probability map is I_2, and the
original head scan is I_3, then the skull stripped image I_S can be obtained by:

$$I_S = I_3. * M \tag{3.2}$$

where M is the mask:

$$M = (I_1 + I_2) > T \tag{3.3}$$

with T being a given threshold.

3.3.3   Other Means

There are other means to carry out skull stripping. 3dSkullStrip is a good program
in Analysis of Functional NeuroImages (AFNI) generated from T_1-weighted MR
images. Scholars also proposed many other excellent approaches. Roura et al. [15]
developed a multispectral adaptive region growing algorithm for axial brain
extraction. Moldovanu et al. [16] proposed a robust skull-stripping method based
on two irrational masks of sizes 3×3 and 5×5 pixels, respectively. Alansary
et al. [17] used linear combination of discrete Gaussians (LCDG) and Markov–
Gibbs random field (MGRF) models to develop an infant brain extraction tool.
Kleesiek et al. [18] developed a deep MRI brain extraction tool via a 3D convolutional neural network (CNN).

3.4   Slice Selection

In pathological brain detection (PBD) systems, each voxel in a volumetric image can be regarded as a feature. Therefore, slice selection is used to select where the lesion or abnormal evidence is located. Slice selection is carried out either by neuroradiologists [19], hardware encoding [20], or algorithms [21]. Note that slice selection is becoming unnecessary since computer processing is becoming faster and therefore cheaper.

Yuan [21] proposed an inter-class variance (ICV) method. They calculated the ICV from the following equation:

$$v(k) = \left\| \mu_p(k) - \mu_h(k) \right\|^2 \tag{3.4}$$

where k is the index of slice; μ_p and μ_h represent the mean of gray-level values of the kth slice of pathological subjects and healthy subjects, respectively; v represents the ICV value; and $\|.\|^2$ represents the l_2-norm [22]. After plotting the curve of ICV value versus slice index, the user can select the slice with maximum ICV values or other specific criteria. Figure 3.9 shows a selected slice from a particular dataset. The ICV values of selected slices should be more than half of the maximum value, and neighboring slices should be separated by 10 further slices.

3.5   Spatial Normalization

The next step in the procedure is spatial normalization (i.e., spatial registration), which reshapes a given brain image to a template image (i.e., reference image) [23]. Two steps are required: (1) estimation of warp field and (2) application of warp field with resampling [24].

Fig. 3.9 Slices selected by ICV

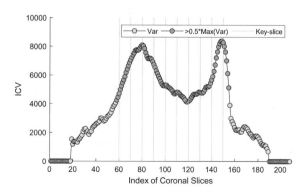

3.5.1 FSL Solution

Usually, brain images are normalized to Montreal Neurological Institute (MNI) space. The FMRIB's linear image registration tool (FLIRT) [25] and non-linear image registration tool (FNIRT) are excellent pieces of software which can accomplish this goal. Figure 3.10 shows a spatially normalized result using FLIRT and FNIRT.

3.5.2 Matlab Solution

The image processing toolbox in Matlab provides registration functions such as:

1. Command "imregister," which can perform intensity based spatial normalization (Table 3.5).
2. Command "imregdemons," which estimates the displacement field that aligns two 2D or 3D images (Table 3.6).

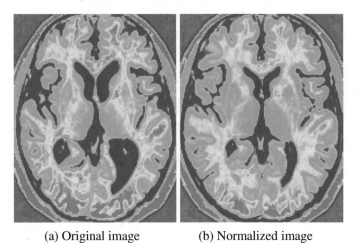

(a) Original image   (b) Normalized image

Fig. 3.10 Spatially normalized image

Table 3.5 The "imregister" command

reg = imregister(moving, fixed, Type, optimizer, metric)
Input moving: moving image fixed: fixed image Type: geometric transformation to be applied to the moving image, including translation, rigid, similarity, affine optimizer: optimization method metric: the similarity metric to be optimized
Output reg: transformed image

Table 3.6 The
"imregdemons" command

[D, reg] = imregdemons (moving, fixed)
Input moving: moving image fixed: fixed image
Output D: displacement field reg: aligned moving image

Besides this, the SPM toolbox can directly help to spatially normalize brain images [26].

Scholars have developed more advanced spatial normalization methods: Lancaster et al. [27] proposed anatomical global spatial normalization methods, in order to scale high-resolution control brains, without altering the mean sizes of brain structures. Rorden et al. [28] introduced specialized templates, which applied normalization algorithms to subjects most likely to suffer strokes due to their age. Li et al. [29] introduced an online spatial normalization method for real-time fMRI. Weiss et al. [30] proposed a multistage system for implementing normalization.

3.6 Intensity Normalization

Intensity normalization or inter-scan normalization has been used to match MR image intensities between MRI scans [31], so as to improve image compatibility and facilitate comparability. Table 3.7 shows four classical intensity normalization methods: intensity scaling [32], histogram stretching [33], Gaussian kernel normalization [34], and histogram normalization [34].

Table 3.7 Intensity normalization methods

Method	Equation
Intensity scaling	$h(x, y) = \dfrac{g(x, y) - g_{hl}}{g_{hh} - g_{hl}}$
Histogram stretching	$h(x, y) = \dfrac{g(x, y) - g_{min}}{g_{max} - g_{min}}$
Gaussian kernel normalization	$h(x, y) = \dfrac{g(x, y) - m_g}{\sigma_g}$
Histogram normalization	$h(x, y) = \dfrac{g_{hh} - g_{hl}}{g_{max} - g_{min}} \times (g(x, y) - g_{min}) + g_{hl}$

Notes g, the original image; h, the intensity normalized image; g_{hh}, the mean value of the homogeneous high-intensity region of interest (ROI); g_{hl}, the mean value of homogeneous low-intensity ROI; g_{min}, the minimum grayscale value; g_{max}, the maximum grayscale value; m_g, the mean of the original image; σ_g, the standard deviation of the original image

3.7   Image Enhancement

Image enhancement is sometimes used in PBD to increase the quality of the brain image. Three basic enhancement methods are: linear, logarithmic, and power-law [35]. Suppose the original image is x and the enhanced image is y, then the logarithmic enhancement is depicted as:

$$y = c \times \log(x + r) \tag{3.5}$$

where r is a non-negative parameter.

The power-law enhancement is depicted as:

$$y = c \times x^r \tag{3.6}$$

This power-law enhancement is also called a gamma correction.

3.7.1   Histogram Equalization

Histogram equalization (HE) [36] adjusts the contrast of the image using a histogram of the original image. Suppose the probability of occurrence of pixels of level i in the original image x is:

$$p_x(i) = \frac{n_i}{n} \tag{3.7}$$

where n is the total number of pixels, and n_i is the total number of pixels with values of i.

We may calculate the cumulative distribution function (CDF) as:

$$c_x(i) = \sum_{j=0}^{i} p_x(j) \tag{3.8}$$

where c represents the CDF.

Then, we create a transformation:

$$y = T(x) \tag{3.9}$$

so that the produced image y can have a histogram with stable amplitude. In this assumption, the CDF of image y should increase linearly with gray-level values as:

$$c_y(i) = i \times K \tag{3.10}$$

where K is a positive parameter. Thus, we have:

$$c_y(T(k)) = c_x(k) \tag{3.11}$$

The Matlab command "histeq" can implement the HE operation, as shown in Table 3.8.

Table 3.8 The "histeq" command	**J = histeq (I, n)**
	Input I: input image n: n discrete gray levels in image J
	Output J: enhanced image

3.7.2   Contrast-Limited Adaptive Histogram Equalization

Contrast-limited adaptive histogram equalization (CLAHE) enhancement is performed on small regions (tiles) within the image rather than the whole image. CLAHE employs bilinear interpolation for combining neighboring tiles without artifacts. Compared to standard histogram equalization methods, CLAHE has three advantages:

1. It uses the histogram of different tiles to redistribute the lightness value of the image.
2. It depresses noise, especially in homogeneous areas.
3. It improves local contrast and enhances edge definition.

Figure 3.11 shows the image enhancement results of a brain image leading to a diagnosis of Herpes encephalitis. It is clear that the enhanced image has better contrast, and that the details in various tissues offer a better visual quality than the original image. The "adapthisteq" command, in Matlab, can implement the CLAHE operation easily, as shown in Table 3.9.

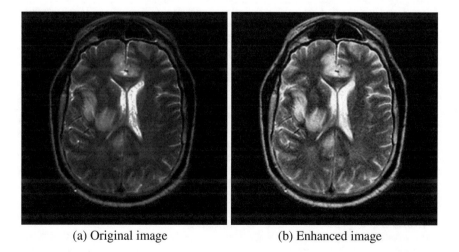

(a) Original image   (b) Enhanced image

Fig. 3.11 Result of CLAHE for a brain image leading to a diagnosis of Herpes encephalitis

Table 3.9 The "adapthisteq" command

J = adapthisteq (I)
Input
I: input image
Output
J: enhanced image

3.8 Conclusion

In this chapter, we have summarized and described the latest image preprocessing techniques, with the aim of performing PBD, identifying the basic steps.

Nevertheless, some steps are not necessary in PBD. The reason for this is analogous to the development of face detection. In traditional face detection, face centering and light variations should be considered. As developments have been made in pattern recognition, these preprocessing methods have become unnecessary in modern face recognition systems.

Yet in our PBD system, some of these preprocessing steps are still essential, removing them would burden subsequent classification performances.

References

1. Keegan J, Gatehouse PD, Taylor AM, Yang GZ, Jhooti P, Firmin DN (1999) Coronary artery imaging in a 0.5-Tesla scanner: Implementation of real-time, navigator echo-controlled segmented k-space FLASH and interleaved-spiral sequences. Magn Reson Med 41(2):392–399
2. Zhu YC, Gao S, Cheng LQ, Bao SL (2013) Review: K-space trajectory development. In: International conference on medical imaging physics and engineering (ICMIPE), Shenyang, P.R. China. IEEE, New York, pp 356–360
3. Peterson BS (2014) Energy preserved sampling for compressed sensing MRI. Comput Math Methods Med, Article ID: 546814. https://doi.org/10.1155/2014/546814
4. Dabek J, Zevenhoven KCJ, Nieminen JO, Vesanen PT, Sepponen R, Ilmoniemi RJ (2012) Gradient-excitation encoding combined with frequency and phase encodings for three-dimensional ultra-low-field MRI. In: Annual international conference of the IEEE Engineering in Medicine and Biology Society, San Diego, CA IEEE Engineering in Medicine and Biology Society conference proceedings. IEEE, New York, pp 1093–1097
5. Wittevrongel B, Van Hulle MM (2016) Frequency- and phase encoded SSVEP using spatiotemporal beamforming. PLoS ONE 11(8), Article ID: e0159988. https://doi.org/10.1371/journal.pone.0159988
6. Wang S, Ji G, Dong Z, Zhang Y (2014) An improved quality guided phase unwrapping method and its applications to MRI. Progress Electromagn Res 145:273–286
7. Ruiz-Antolin D, Segura J (2016) A new type of sharp bounds for ratios of modified Bessel functions. J Math Anal Appl 443(2):1232–1246. https://doi.org/10.1016/j.jmaa.2016.06.011

8. Iftikhar MA, Jalil A, Rathore S, Hussain M (2014) Robust brain MRI denoising and segmentation using enhanced non-local means algorithm. Int J Imaging Syst Technol 24 (1):52–66

9. Phophalia A, Rajwade A, Mitra SK (2014) Rough set based image denoising for brain MR images. Sig Process 103:24–35. https://doi.org/10.1016/j.sigpro.2014.01.029

10. Yang J, Fan JF, Ai DN, Zhou SJ, Tang SY, Wang YT (2015) Brain MR image denoising for Rician noise using pre-smooth non-local means filter. Biomed Eng Online 14, Article ID: 2. https://doi.org/10.1186/1475-925x-14-2

11. Phophalia A, Mitra SK (2015) Rough set based bilateral filter design for denoising brain MR images. Appl Soft Comput 33:1–14. https://doi.org/10.1016/j.asoc.2015.04.005

12. Akar SA (2016) Determination of optimal parameters for bilateral filter in brain MR image denoising. Appl Soft Comput 43:87–96. https://doi.org/10.1016/j.asoc.2016.02.043

13. Kalavathi P, Prasath VBS (2016) Methods on skull stripping of MRI head scan images—a review. J Digit Imaging 29(3):365–379. https://doi.org/10.1007/s10278-015-9847-8

14. Smith SM (2002) Fast robust automated brain extraction. Hum Brain Mapp 17(3):143–155. https://doi.org/10.1002/hbm.10062

15. Roura E, Oliver A, Cabezas M, Vilanova JC, Rovira A, Ramio-Torrenta L, Llado X (2014) MARGA: Multispectral Adaptive Region Growing Algorithm for brain extraction on axial MRI. Comput Methods Programs Biomed 113(2):655–673. https://doi.org/10.1016/j.cmpb.2013.11.015

16. Moldovanu S, Moraru L, Biswas A (2015) Robust skull-stripping segmentation based on irrational mask for magnetic resonance brain images. J Digit Imaging 28(6):738–747. https://doi.org/10.1007/s10278-015-9776-6

17. Alansary A, Ismail M, Soliman A, Khalifa F, Nitzken M, Elnakib A, Mostapha M, Black A, Stinebruner K, Casanova MF, Zurada JM, El-Baz A (2016) Infant brain extraction in T1-weighted MR images using BET and refinement using LCDG and MGRF models. IEEE J Biomed Health Inf 20(3):925–935. https://doi.org/10.1109/jbhi.2015.2415477

18. Kleesiek J, Urban G, Hubert A, Schwarz D, Maier-Hein K, Bendszus M, Biller A (2016) Deep MRI brain extraction: A 3D convolutional neural network for skull stripping. Neuroimage 129:460–469. https://doi.org/10.1016/j.neuroimage.2016.01.024

19. Mirsadraee S, Tse M, Kershaw L, Semple S, Schembri N, Chin C, Murchison JT, Hirani N, van Beek EJR (2016) T1 characteristics of interstitial pulmonary fibrosis on 3T MRI: a predictor of early interstitial change? Quant Imaging Med Surgery 6(1):42–49. https://doi.org/10.3978/j.issn.2223-4292.2016.02.02

20. Middione MJ, Thompson RB, Ennis DB (2014) Velocity encoding with the slice select refocusing gradient for faster imaging and reduced chemical shift-induced phase errors. Magn Reson Med 71(6):2014–2023. https://doi.org/10.1002/mrm.24861

21. Yuan TF (2015) Detection of subjects and brain regions related to Alzheimer's disease using 3D MRI scans based on eigenbrain and machine learning. Front Comput Neurosci 9, Article ID: 66. https://doi.org/10.3389/fncom.2015.00066

22. Wang S-H (2016) Single slice based detection for Alzheimer's disease via wavelet entropy and multilayer perceptron trained by biogeography-based optimization. Multimed Tools Appl. https://doi.org/10.1007/s11042-016-4222-4

23. Buchholz HG, Pfeifer P, Miederer M, Fehr C, Schreckenberger M (2015) Impact of different strategies on spatial normalization of F-18-fallypride: head-to-head comparison of MRI-based and PET-based methods. J Nucl Med 56(3):1–11

24. Kronfeld A, Buchholz HG, Maus S, Reuss S, Muller-Forell W, Lutz B, Schreckenberger M, Miederer I (2015) Evaluation of MRI and cannabinoid type 1 receptor PET templates constructed using DARTEL for spatial normalization of rat brains. Med Phys 42(12):6875–6884. https://doi.org/10.1118/1.4934825

25. Jenkinson M, Bannister P, Brady M, Smith S (2002) Improved optimization for the robust and accurate linear registration and motion correction of brain images. Neuroimage 17(2):825–841. https://doi.org/10.1006/nimg.2002.1132

26. Rosario BL, Ziolko SK, Weissfeld LA, Price JC (2008) Assessment of parameter settings for SPM5 spatial normalization of structural MRI data: application to type 2 diabetes. Neuroimage 41(2):363–370. https://doi.org/10.1016/j.neuroimage.2008.02.004

27. Lancaster JL, Cykowski MD, McKay DR, Kochunov PV, Fox PT, Rogers W, Toga AW, Zilles K, Amunts K, Mazziotta J (2010) Anatomical global spatial normalization. Neuroinformatics 8(3):171–182. https://doi.org/10.1007/s12021-010-9074-x

28. Rorden C, Bonilha L, Fridriksson J, Bender B, Karnath HO (2012) Age-specific CT and MRI templates for spatial normalization. Neuroimage 61(4):957–965. https://doi.org/10.1016/j.neuroimage.2012.03.020

29. Li XF, Yao L, Ye Q, Zhao XJ (2014) Online spatial normalization for real-time fMRI. PLoS ONE 9 (7), Article ID: e103302. https://doi.org/10.1371/journal.pone.0103302

30. Weiss M, Alkemade A, Keuken MC, Muller-Axt C, Geyer S, Turner R, Forstmann BU (2015) Spatial normalization of ultrahigh resolution 7 T magnetic resonance imaging data of the postmortem human subthalamic nucleus: a multistage approach. Brain Struct Funct 220 (3):1695–1703. https://doi.org/10.1007/s00429-014-0754-4

31. Zhan T (2016) Pathological brain detection by artificial intelligence in magnetic resonance imaging scanning. Progress Electromagn Res 156:105–133

32. Abbott DF, Pell GS, Pardoe H, Jackson GD (2009) Voxel-Based Iterative Sensitivity (VBIS) analysis: MEthods and a validation of intensity scaling for T2-weighted imaging of hippocampal sclerosis. Neuroimage 44(3):812–819. https://doi.org/10.1016/j.neuroimage.2008.09.055

33. Brahim A, Gorriz JM, Ramirez J, Khedher L (2015) Intensity normalization of DaTSCAN SPECT imaging using a model-based clustering approach. Appl Soft Comput 37:234–244. https://doi.org/10.1016/j.asoc.2015.08.030

34. Loizou GP, Pantziaris M, Pattichis CS, Seimenis I (2013) Brain MR image normalization in texture analysis of multiple sclerosis. J Biomed Graph Comput 3(1):20–30

35. Dong Z (2016) Simulation of digital image processing in medical applications. SIMULATION 92(9):825–826

36. Amil FM, Rahman S, Rahman MM, Dey EK (2016) Bilateral histogram equalization for contrast enhancement. Int J Softw Innov 4(4):15–34. https://doi.org/10.4018/ijsi.2016100102

Chapter 4
Canonical Feature Extraction Methods for Structural Magnetic Resonance Imaging

Handcrafted features play an important role in PBD systems. In this chapter, some widely used features, used in PBD, are introduced. First, common 2D and 3D shape features are presented. Then, statistical measures (mean, variance, standard deviation, median, skewness, and kurtosis) and statistical plots (radar chart, pie chart, bar chart, wind rose, etc.) are discussed. The development of image moments is given, from raw moments, to central moments, to normalized central moments, to Hu moments. Besides this, a comparison between a Zernike moment and pseudo Zernike moment is provided. Gray-level co-occurrence matrix and Haralick features are discussed. Further, the standard Fourier transform, and its two important variants (sine and cosine transform), are explained. The fractional Fourier transform, and its three fast discrete implementation methods, are presented. Finally, three important entropy features are compared, i.e., Shannon entropy, Tsallis entropy, and Renyi entropy. Readers will see, in subsequent chapters, that most brain feature extraction methods practically used are in fact combinations of simple features introduced in this chapter.

4.1 Shape Feature

Physicians and neuroradiologists prefer to use shape features for specified brain tissues, since they have strong physiological meaning, as shown in Fig. 4.1.

Shape features are extracted from the lobes (frontal lobe, parietal lobe, occipital lobe, temporal lobe, and limbic lobe), brain stem (medullar, pons, and midbrain), diencephalon, cerebellum, ventricles (lateral ventricles, third ventricle, fourth ventricle), tracts, vessels (arteries and veins), and even the whole brain. Figure 4.2 presents a rough segmentation of a human brain.

Tables 4.1 and 4.2 list 2D and 3D shape features, respectively. 2D shape features include perimeter, arc length, area, eccentricity, distance, etc. 3D shape features include surface area, volume, girth, distance, etc.

© Springer Nature Singapore Pte Ltd. 2018
S.-H. Wang et al., *Pathological Brain Detection*, Brain Informatics and Health,
https://doi.org/10.1007/978-981-10-4026-9_4

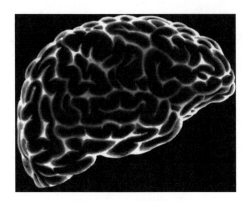

Fig. 4.1 The brain can be viewed as a combination of shapes

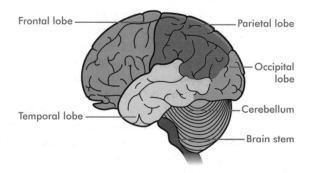

Fig. 4.2 A rough segmentation of the brain

Table 4.1 2D shape features

Shape	Definition
Perimeter/circumference	Length of the outline of a shape
Arc length	Length of an irregular arc segment
Area	Extent of a 2D shape
Eccentricity	How much the conic section deviates from being circular
Distance	How far apart objects are

Table 4.2 3D shape features

Shape	Definition
Surface area	Total area that the surface of the object occupies
Volume	The 3D space an object occupies
Girth	The perimeter of an object projected along a certain direction
Distance	How far apart objects are

Besides this, a convex polygon is often used, which is defined as a simple polygon in which no line segment between two points on the boundary of the brain tissue goes outside this polygon. The properties of this polygon are usually used to represent the shape features of brain tissue.

4.2 Statistical Measure

Statistical measures are based on spatial pixels [1].

4.2.1 Common Measures

Consider pixels $\{x\}$ as the possible values of a discrete random variable X associated with a particular probability distribution P. We can then define common statistical measures including mean, variance, standard deviation, median, skewness, and kurtosis. Table 4.3 gives the meaning of these statistical measures.

These seven measures are defined below. The mean μ is defined as:

$$\mu = \mathrm{E}(x) \tag{4.1}$$

The variance V is defined as:

$$V = \mathrm{E}\left[(x - \mu)^2\right] \tag{4.2}$$

The standard deviation σ is defined as:

$$\sigma = \sqrt{\mathrm{E}\left[(x - \mu)^2\right]} \tag{4.3}$$

Table 4.3 Meanings of statistical measures

Measure	Meaning
Mean	Expectation of central tendency
Variance	Expectation of squared deviation from the mean
Standard deviation	Variation of the dataset
Median	The value separating the higher half from the lower half
Skewness	Asymmetry of probability function from the mean
Kurtosis	Tailedness of the probability function

Measure	Matlab command
Mean	M = mean (A)
Variance	V = var (A)
Standard deviation	S = std (A)
Median	M = median (A)
Skewness	y = skewness (A)
Kurtosis	k = kurtosis (A)

Table 4.4 Matlab commands for common statistical measures

The median m is defined as:

$$m : P(x \leq m) = P(x \geq m) = \frac{1}{2} \tag{4.4}$$

The skewness s is defined as:

$$s = E\left(\frac{x - \mu}{\sigma}\right)^3 \tag{4.5}$$

The kurtosis k is defined as:

$$k = \frac{E\left[(x - \mu)^4\right]}{\left\{E\left[(x - \mu)^2\right]\right\}^2} \tag{4.6}$$

In Matlab, the functions for these statistical measures are illustrated in Table 4.4.

4.2.2   Statistical Chart

Figure 4.3 presents several types of commonly used statistical graphs, including radar charts, pie charts, bar charts, wind roses, etc.

- A radar chart can display multivariate data in a 2D plane. It is also called a web chart, spider chart [2], star chart, cobweb chart, Kiviat diagram, etc.
- A pie chart gives a circular statistical graphic that is segmented into slices to illustrate numerical proportion. It is also called a circle chart.
- A bar chart shows grouped data with rectangular bars, whose lengths are proportional to their corresponding values.
- A wind rose plot was originally used by meteorologists to give a succinct view of wind speed and direction.

Fig. 4.3 Several commonly used statistical graphs

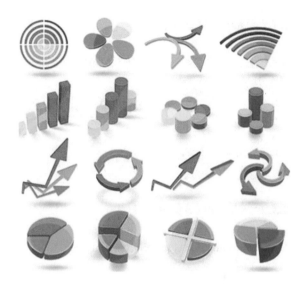

4.3 Image Moments

Image shape feature plays a very fundamental role in image classification, so effective and efficient shape descriptors are a key component of image representation [3]. We use an image moment as the shape descriptor. The development of an image moment is shown in Fig. 4.4.

Fig. 4.4 Development of an image moment

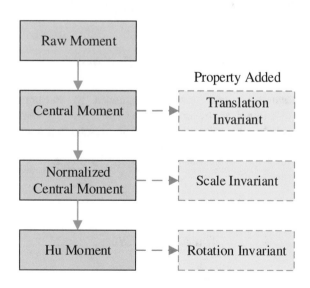

4.3.1   Raw Moments

For an magnetic resonance (MR) brain image $I(x, y)$, the raw moment [4] of order $(p + q)$ is defined as:

$$M_{pq} = \sum_{x} \sum_{y} x^p y^q I(x, y) \tag{4.7}$$

where $p, q = 0, 1, 2, \ldots$

4.3.2   Central Moments

A central moment μ is usually used in real applications to replace the raw moment in Eq. (4.7).

$$\mu_{pq} = \sum_{x} \sum_{y} (x - \bar{x})^p (y - \bar{y})^q I(x, y) \tag{4.8}$$

$$\bar{x} = \frac{M_{10}}{M_{00}} \tag{4.9}$$

$$\bar{y} = \frac{M_{01}}{M_{00}} \tag{4.10}$$

Central moments are translational-invariant.

4.3.3   Normalized Central Moments

Central moments can be extended to be both translational-invariant and scale-invariant, by dividing the corresponding central moment by the properly scaled (00)th moment. The division results in a normalized central moment.

$$\eta_{pq} = \frac{\mu_{pq}}{\mu_{00}^{\left(\frac{p+q}{2}+1\right)}} \tag{4.11}$$

4.3.4   Hu Moment Invariants

To enable invariance to rotation, the moments mentioned above require further reformulation. Hu [5] described two different methods for producing rotation moment invariants.

It was noted that the first method, called principal axes, can break down when images do not have unique principal axes. Such images are described as being rotationally symmetric [6].

The second method is the Hu moment invariant (HMI) method. Hu derived these expressions from algebraic invariants applied to the moment-generating function under a rotational transformation [7]. They consist of a set of nonlinear centralized moment expressions:

$$H_1 = \eta_{20} + \eta_{02} \tag{4.12}$$

$$H_2 = (\eta_{20} - \eta_{02})^2 + 4\eta_{11}^2 \tag{4.13}$$

$$H_3 = (\eta_{30} - 3\eta_{12})^2 + (3\eta_{21} - \eta_{03})^2 \tag{4.14}$$

$$H_4 = (\eta_{30} + \eta_{12})^2 + (\eta_{21} + \eta_{03})^2 \tag{4.15}$$

$$H_5 = (\eta_{30} - 3\eta_{12})(\eta_{30} + \eta_{12})\left[(\eta_{30} + \eta_{12})^2 - 3(\eta_{21} + \eta_{03})^2\right] \\ + (3\eta_{21} - \eta_{03})(\eta_{21} + \eta_{03})\left[3(\eta_{30} + \eta_{12})^2 - (\eta_{21} + \eta_{03})^2\right] \tag{4.16}$$

$$H_6 = (\eta_{20} - \eta_{02})\left[(\eta_{30} + \eta_{12})^2 - (\eta_{21} + \eta_{03})\right]^2 \\ + 4\eta_{11}(\eta_{30} + \eta_{12})(\eta_{21} + \eta_{03}) \tag{4.17}$$

$$H_7 = (3\eta_{21} - \eta_{03})(\eta_{30} + \eta_{12})\left[(\eta_{30} + \eta_{12})^2 - 3(\eta_{21} + \eta_{03})^2\right] \\ - (\eta_{30} - 3\eta_{12})(\eta_{21} + \eta_{03})\left[3(\eta_{30} + \eta_{12})^2 - (\eta_{21} + \eta_{03})^2\right] \tag{4.18}$$

It is clearly observed that HMI is a set of absolute orthogonal (i.e., rotational) moment invariants [8], which can be used for scale, translation, and rotation invariant pattern identification.

4.4 Zernike Moments

Zernike moments (ZMs) have gained great success in many fields. Tahmasbi et al. [9] employed ZMs to classify benign and malignant masses in mammography diagnosis systems. Sharma and Khanna [10] developed a computer-aided diagnosis of malignant mammograms using ZMs and a support vector machine (SVM). Farokhi et al. [11] employed ZMs and Hermite kernels to recognize near-infrared facial images.

4.4.1   Basic Form of Zernike Moments

Zernike polynomials (ZPs) are orthogonal on a unit disk (the set points whose distance from the origin is less than 1). Suppose φ represents the azimuth angle and ρ represents the radial distance within the range [0, 1]. ZPs are defined as:

$$V_n^m(\rho, \varphi) = R_n^m(\rho) \exp(jm\varphi) \tag{4.19}$$

where V represents a ZP; n (a non-negative integer) represents the order; m (an integer) represents the repetition, with the restrain of $n \geq |m|$ and $n - m$ as even. R_n^m represents the radial polynomial defined as:

$$R_n^m(\rho) = \sum_{k=0}^{\frac{n-m}{2}} \frac{(-1)^k (n-k)!}{k!(\frac{n+m}{2} - k)!(\frac{n-m}{2} - k)!} \rho^{n-2k} \tag{4.20}$$

Since ZPs are orthogonal to each other, they are widely used as base functions of image moments. The ZMs can represent global image characteristics, without information redundancy. Another advantage of a ZM is that its magnitude is independent to the rotation angle; hence, it is extremely well suited for describing the shape features of an image.

4.4.2   Pseudo Zernike Moment

A ZP contains only $(n + 1)(n + 2)/2$ linear and orthogonal polynomials, which limits its applications. Pseudo Zernike polynomials (PZPs) [12] were proposed, so as to generate more features with numbers of $(n + 1)^2$. Besides this, pseudo Zernike moments (PZMs) are more robust than ZMs and less sensitive to image noise than ZMs [13]. Their difference lies in the radial polynomials that are given real values [14]. Mathematically, PZPs are defined with following form [15]:

$$Z_n^m(\rho, \varphi) = D_n^m(\rho) \exp(jm\varphi) \tag{4.21}$$

Here $|m| \leq n$. The radial polynomials D_n^m are defined as:

$$D_n^m(\rho) = \sum_{k=0}^{n-m} \frac{(-1)^k (2n+1-k)!}{k!(n+m-k+1)!(n-m-k)!} \rho^{n-k} \tag{4.22}$$

Fast calculations of ZMs and PZMs can be found in [16].

Fig. 4.5 Relationship
between Cartesian and polar
coordinates

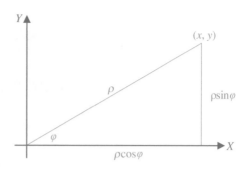

4.4.3 Coordinate Transform

To extract ZMs or PZMs from a given image $I(x, y)$, we need to transform between
Cartesian and polar coordinates [17], as shown in Fig. 4.5. The mathematical
formula for this is:

$$x = \rho \cos \varphi$$
$$y = \rho \sin \varphi$$

(4.23)

Then, the ZMs and PZMs of $I(x, y)$ are obtained by following equations:

$$ZM = \frac{n+1}{\pi} \sum_x \sum_y I(x,y) \left[V_n^m(x,y) \right]^*$$

(4.24)

$$PZM = \frac{n+1}{\pi} \sum_x \sum_y I(x,y) \left[R_n^m(x,y) \right]^*$$

(4.25)

4.4.4 Illustration of Pseudo Zernike Polynomials

Figure 4.6 illustrates pseudo Zernike polynomials (PZPs) with a maximum order
$n = 6$. For $n = 0$, we have only one PZP of Z_0^0. For $n = 1$, we have three PZPs of
Z_1^{-1}, Z_1^0, and Z_1^1. For $n = 2$, we have five PZPs. The PZP and total number at $n = 3$,
4, 5, and 6 are listed in Table 4.5.

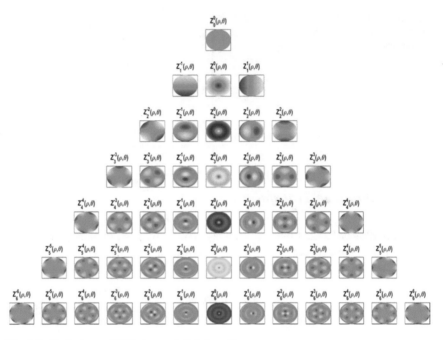

Fig. 4.6 Illustrations of PZPs in a unit disk ($n = 6$)

Table 4.5 PZPs for each order

Order	PZP	Number
$n = 0$	Z_0^0	1
$n = 1$	Z_1^{-1}, Z_1^0, Z_1^1	3
$n = 2$	$Z_2^{-2}, Z_2^{-1}, Z_2^0, Z_2^1, Z_2^2$	5
$n = 3$	$Z_3^{-3}, Z_3^{-2}, Z_3^{-1}, Z_3^0, Z_3^1, Z_3^2, Z_3^3$	7
$n = 4$	$Z_4^{-4}, Z_4^{-3}, Z_4^{-2}, Z_4^{-1}, Z_4^0, Z_4^1, Z_4^2, Z_4^3, Z_4^4$	9
$n = 5$	$Z_5^{-5}, Z_5^{-4}, Z_5^{-3}, Z_5^{-2}, Z_5^{-1}, Z_5^0, Z_5^1, Z_5^2, Z_5^3, Z_5^4, Z_5^5$	11
$n = 6$	$Z_6^{-6}, Z_6^{-5}, Z_6^{-4}, Z_6^{-3}, Z_6^{-2}, Z_6^{-1}, Z_6^0, Z_6^1, Z_6^2, Z_6^3, Z_6^4, Z_6^5, Z_6^6$	13

4.5 Gray-Level Co-occurrence Matrix

A gray-level co-occurrence matrix (GLCM) is defined to be a distribution of co-occurring values at a given offset over a brain image [18]. Suppose an image is represented as I, its offset being (Δx, Δy), then the GLCM of the image is defined as:

$$G_{\Delta x, \Delta y}(i,j) = \sum_x \sum_y \begin{cases} 1 & \text{if } I(x,y) = i \text{ and } I(x+\Delta x, y+\Delta y) = j \\ 0 & \text{otherwise} \end{cases} \quad (4.26)$$

where G is the co-occurrence matrix and i and j are the image intensity values. The offset makes GLCM sensitive to rotation [19], hence the offsets in practical are chosen as $0°$, $45°$, $90°$, and $135°$ at an identical distance to achieve rotational invariance [20].

Three famous implementation methods are shown in Table 4.6. First, using the Matlab platform, we can use the command "graycomatrix" to create a GLCM from an image, and use "graycoprops" to extract 4 properties, i.e., contrast, correlation, energy, and homogeneity from it [21]. Second, using R language, the "glcm" package [22] can be used to obtain 8 features, i.e., mean, variance, homogeneity, contrast, dissimilarity, entropy, second moment, and correlation. Third, Haralick and Shanmugam [23] presented in total 14 Haralick features with the intent of describing the texture of an image.

In particular we will analyze the two commands in Matlab. The details of the "graycomatrix" and "graycoprops" commands are given in Tables 4.7 and 4.8, respectively.

Table 4.6 Comparison of three variants of GLCM features

GLCM variants	Content
Matlab-generated features	Contrast, correlation, energy, and homogeneity
R-generated features	Mean, variance, homogeneity, contrast, dissimilarity, entropy, second moment, and correlation
Haralick features	Angular second moment, contrast, correlation, sum of squared variances, inverse difference moment, sum average, sum variance, sum entropy, entropy, difference variance, difference entropy, information measures of correlation 1 and 2, and maximal correlation coefficient

Table 4.7 The "graycomatrix" command

glcms = graycomatrix(I)
Input I: input image
Output glcms: The GLCM matrices

Table 4.8 The
"graycoprops" command

stats = graycoprops(glcm, properties)
Input
glcm: The GLCM matrices
properties: any combination of contrast, correlation, energy, and homogeneity
Output
stats: The statistical output

4.6 Fourier Transform

A Fourier transform (FT) decomposes a signal into the frequency domain that
makes it up [24]. For brain images, a discrete Fourier transform (DFT) is normally
used which converts the image into a finite combination of complex sinusoids
ordered by frequency.

4.6.1 Discrete Fourier Transform

Suppose signal X is composed of N complex numbers of $[x_0, x_1, \ldots, x_{N-1}]$, the DFT
is defined as:

$$X_k = \sum_{n=0}^{N-1} x_n \times \exp\left(-\frac{2\pi ikn}{N}\right) \tag{4.27}$$

The fast Fourier transform (FFT) can reduce the computing complexity in the
DFT of $O(N^2)$ to $O(N\log N)$. Figure 4.7 shows the frequency domain of a random
generated signal.

4.6.2 Discrete Sine and Cosine Transform

In some conditions, sines and cosines are used to replace complex numbers,
yielding the discrete sine transform (DST) [25] and discrete cosine transform
(DCT) [26]:

$$\text{DST} : X_k = \sum_{n=0}^{N-1} x_n \times \sin\left[\frac{\pi}{N+1}(n+1)(k+1)\right] \tag{4.28}$$

$$\text{DCT} : X_k = \sum_{n=0}^{N-1} x_n \times \cos\left[\frac{\pi}{N}\left(n+\frac{1}{2}\right)k\right] \tag{4.29}$$

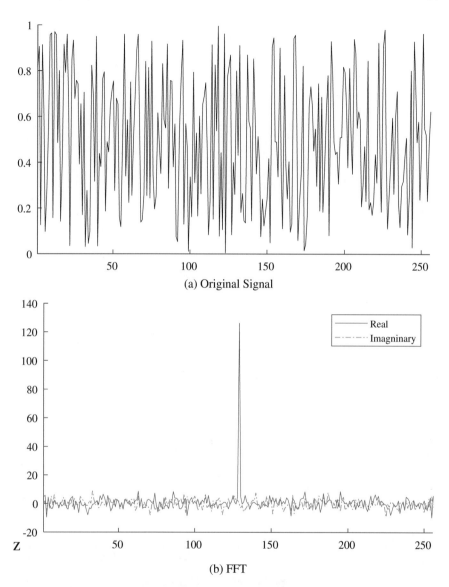

Fig. 4.7 An illustration of discrete Fourier transform

For better vision and understanding, Fig. 4.8 shows DST and DCT decomposition.

In all, the DFT, DST, and DCT, and their inverse transforms, can be implemented using simple commands in Matlab, as shown in Table 4.9. The 2D version is shown in Table 4.10—note that commands "dst" and "idst" do not have corresponding 2D versions.

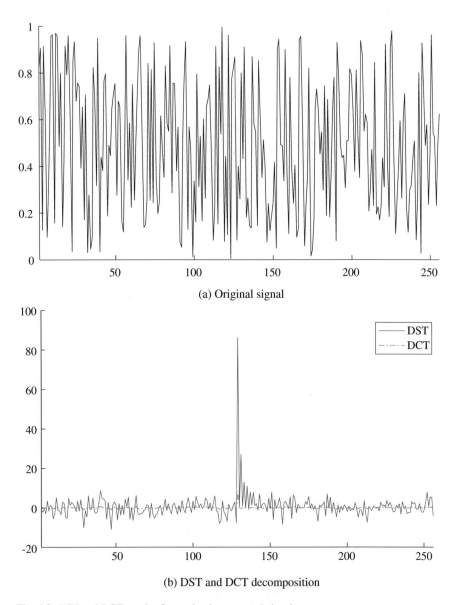

(a) Original signal

(b) DST and DCT decomposition

Fig. 4.8 DST and DCT result of a randomly generated signal

	Transform	Matlab code
Table 4.9 Codes for 1D DFT, DST, and DCT	DFT	y = fft(x)
	Inverse DFT	x = ifft(y)
	DST	y = dst(x)
	Inverse DST	x = idst(y)
	DCT	y = dct(x)
	Inverse DCT	x = idct(y)

	Transform	Matlab code
Table 4.10 Codes for 2D DFT and DCT	DFT	y = fft2(x)
	Inverse DFT	x = ifft2(y)
	DCT	y = dct2(x)
	Inverse DCT	x = idct2(y)

4.7 Fractional Fourier Transform

Fractional Fourier transform (FRFT) [27] introduces a new angle parameter α, which represents the rotational angle in the time–frequency domain. The α-angle transformation of a signal $x(t)$ is:

$$X_\alpha(u) = \int_{-\infty}^{\infty} K_\alpha(t,u)x(t)\,dt \qquad (4.30)$$

where u represents the frequency and K the FRFT transformation kernel as:

$$K_\alpha(t,u) = \sqrt{1 - i \cot \alpha}\ \exp\big(i\pi(t^2 \cot \alpha - 2ut \csc \alpha + u^2 \cot \alpha)\big) \qquad (4.31)$$

where i is the imaginary unit. The cot and csc functions will diverge if α is a multiple of π. This can be dealt with limits:

$$K_\alpha(t,u) = \begin{cases} \sqrt{1 - i \cot \alpha} \times \exp(i\pi(t^2 \cot \alpha - 2ut \csc \alpha + u^2 \cot \alpha)) \\ \delta(t+u) \\ \delta(t-u) \end{cases},$$

$$\text{for } \alpha \begin{cases} \neq n\pi \\ = (2n+1)\pi \\ = 2n\pi \end{cases} \qquad (4.32)$$

where n is an arbitrary integer and δ the Dirac delta function.

4.7.1 Unified Time–Frequency Domain

For a 1D time signal, a FRFT transforms the signal in time domain to a "unified time–frequency domain (UTFD)" [28]. Figure 4.9 takes a triangular signal as an example and gives UTFD representations with different angles from 0 to 1.

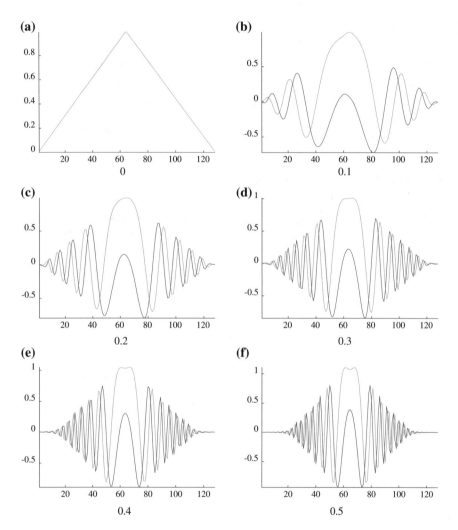

Fig. 4.9 UTFD (green represents the real part, blue the imaginary part, *x* axis represent time domain, and *y* axis represent amplitude)

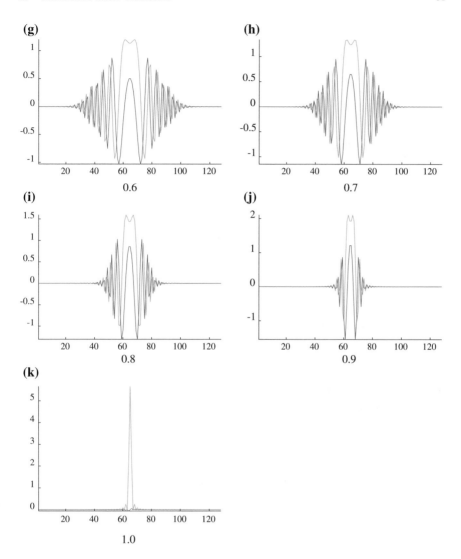

Fig. 4.9 (continued)

4.7.2   Weighted-Type Fractional Fourier Transform

The discrete fractional Fourier transform (DFRFT) is the discrete version of the FRFT. Currently, there are three popular methods for its calculation [29]. Weighted-type FRFT (also known as 4-weighted FRFT, 4-WFRFT, weighted FRFT, and WFRFT) is the simplest, replacing the continuous variables t and u with their discrete versions n and k, respectively. It is defined in following form [30, 31]:

$$F_\alpha = \sum_{i=0}^{3} a_i(\alpha) F_i \tag{4.33}$$

$$a_i(\alpha) = \frac{1}{4} \sum_{k=1}^{4} \exp\left[i\left(\alpha - i\frac{\pi}{2}\right)k\right] \tag{4.34}$$

where F is the Fourier transform. The definition of F_i is:

$$F_k = (F)^k \tag{4.35}$$

Particularly:

$$F_2 = P \tag{4.36}$$

$$F_3 = F_{-1} \tag{4.37}$$

$$F_4 = F_0 = I \tag{4.38}$$

where P is the parity operator (flips the signal function or inverts the time) and I the identity operator.

It is clear from Eq. (4.33) that this definition is the linear weighted combination of the identity matrix, DFT matrix, time inverse matrix, and inverse DFT (IDFT) matrix [32]. It obeys the rotation principle of the FRFT, and it can be computed through a fast algorithm. However, it does not provide transforms similar to those of the FRFT [33].

4.7.3 Sampling-Type Fractional Fourier Transform

Ozaktas et al. [33] provided an algorithm for the efficient and accurate computation of FRFT in O(Nlog$N$) time. The sample-type FRFT of $x(t)$ was defined as:

$$X_\alpha(u) = A_\phi \int_{-\infty}^{\infty} \exp\left(i\pi(t^2 \cot\phi - 2tt' \csc\phi + t'^2 \cot\phi)\right) x(t')\mathrm{d}t' \tag{4.39}$$

where

$$A_\phi = \frac{\exp(-i\pi\mathrm{sgn}(\sin\phi)/4 + i\phi/2)}{|\sin\phi|^{1/2}} \tag{4.40}$$

where

$$\phi = \alpha\pi/2 \tag{4.41}$$

They broke down the FRFT into a chirp multiplication followed by a chirp convolution followed by another chirp multiplication. We will now discuss this three-step approach in detail.

First, multiply the signal $x(t)$ with a chirp function, resulting in $g(t)$:

$$g(t) = x(t)\exp\left(-i\pi t^2 \tan\frac{\phi}{2}\right) \tag{4.42}$$

The bandwidth of $g(t)$ is twice that of $x(t)$. The samples of $g(t)$ are required at intervals of $1/(2\Delta x)$ if the sample interval of $x(t)$ is $1/\Delta x$. Therefore, $g(t)$ is obtained by interpolating $x(t)$ and then multiplying it by the samples of the chirp function.

Second, convolve $g(t)$ with a chirp function and obtain:

$$g'(t) = A_\phi \int_{-\infty}^{\infty} g(t')\exp\left(i\pi(t-t')^2 \csc\phi\right)dt' \tag{4.43}$$

To perform this convolution more efficiently, the chirp function can be replaced with its band-limited version since $g(t)$ is also band-limited:

$$g'(t) = A_\phi \int_{-\infty}^{\infty} h(t-t')g(t')\,dt' \tag{4.44}$$

where

$$h(t) = \int_{-\Delta t}^{\Delta t} H(v)\exp\left(i2\pi vt\right)dv \tag{4.45}$$

where

$$H(v) = \frac{1}{\sqrt{\csc\phi}}\exp(i\pi/4)\exp\left(-\frac{i\pi v^2}{\csc\phi}\right) \tag{4.46}$$

Therefore, Eq. (4.43) can be sampled as:

$$g'\left(\frac{m}{2\Delta x}\right) = \sum_{n=-N}^{N} h\left(\frac{m-n}{2\Delta x}\right)g\left(\frac{n}{2\Delta x}\right) \tag{4.47}$$

Third, another chirp multiplication is performed as:

$$X_\alpha(u) = \exp\left(-i\pi u^2 \tan(\phi/2)\right)g'(u) \tag{4.48}$$

We obtain samples X_α which are spaced at $1/(2\Delta x)$. Since all transforms of x (t) are band-limited to the interval $[-\Delta x/2, \Delta x/2]$, we decimate these samples by a factor of 2 to obtain samples spaced at $1/\Delta x$.

4.7.4 Eigendecomposition-Type Fractional Fourier Transform

The eigendecomposition-type FRFT is generated on the basis that the power of the matrix can be calculated from its eigendecomposition, and directly obtained by the powers of the eigenvalues. The eigendecomposition, i.e., spectral expansion, is firstly used to define the FRFT [34].

Pei and Yeh [35] first suggested this eigendecomposition type of DFRFT, which defined the transform kernel of the DFRFT by taking the fractional powers of the eigenvalues:

$$
F_{2\alpha/\pi} = VD^{2\alpha/\pi}V^{\mathrm{T}}
$$

$$
= \begin{cases}
\displaystyle\sum_{k=0}^{N-1} \exp(-ik\alpha)v_k v_k^{\mathrm{T}} & N \text{ odd} \\[4mm]
\displaystyle\left(\sum_{k=0}^{N-2} \exp\left(-ik\alpha\right)v_k v_k^{\mathrm{T}}\right) + \exp(-iN\alpha)v_{N-1}v_{N-1}^{\mathrm{T}} & N \text{ even}
\end{cases} \tag{4.49}
$$

where v_k represents the eigenvector obtained from matrix S; v_k has k sign changes in the DFT-shifted case; and $V = [v_0|v_1|\dots|v_{N-1}]$.

D is a diagonal matrix, in which the diagonal entries have the same eigenvalues corresponding to the column eigenvectors of matrix V. The form of S is defined as [36]:

$$
S = \begin{bmatrix}
2 & 1 & 0 & 0 & \dots & 0 & 1 \\
1 & 2\cos\omega & 1 & 0 & \dots & 0 & 0 \\
0 & 1 & 2\cos 2\omega & 1 & \dots & 0 & 0 \\
\vdots & \vdots & \vdots & & \ddots & \vdots & \vdots \\
1 & 0 & 0 & 0 & \dots & 1 & 2\cos(N-1)\omega
\end{bmatrix} \tag{4.50}
$$

where $\omega = 2\pi/N$.

Fig. 4.10 Entropy was
developed from
thermodynamics

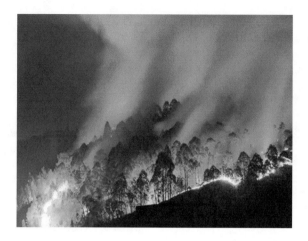

4.8 Entropy

In statistical thermodynamics, entropy is a measure of the number of microscopic configurations which correspond to a thermodynamic system as shown in Fig. 4.10.

Entropy has now been introduced to the field of information theory and is used to measure the information contained in a specific message.

4.8.1 Shannon Entropy

Shannon redefined the entropy concept of Boltzmann/Gibbs as a measure of uncertainty regarding the information content of a system [37]. Shannon entropy is defined from the probability distribution, where p_i denotes the probability of each state i. Therefore, Shannon entropy can be described as:

$$S = -\sum_{i=1}^{L} p_i \log_2(p_i) \tag{4.51}$$

where L denotes the total number of states.

Shannon entropy can be implemented by the "entropy" command in Matlab, as detailed in Table 4.11.

Table 4.11 The "entropy" command

E = entropy(I)
Input
I: input image
Output
E: entropy value

The FRFT can be combined with Shannon entropy to form a new feature of fractional Fourier entropy [38–40].

4.8.2 Tsallis Entropy

Shannon entropy is restricted to the domain of validity of Boltzmann–Gibbs–Shannon (BGS) statistics, which only describes nature when the effective microscopic interactions and the microscopic memory are short ranged [41].

Suppose a physical system can be decomposed into two statistically independent subsystems A and B, Shannon entropy has the extensive property (additivity):

$$S(A+B) = S(A) + S(B) \tag{4.52}$$

Nevertheless, for a certain class of physical systems that entails long-range interactions, long-term memory, and fractal-type structures, it is necessary to use non-extensive entropy. Tsallis [42] proposed a generalization of BGS statistics—its form can be depicted as:

$$S_q = \frac{1 - \sum_{i=1}^{q} (p_i)^q}{q-1} \tag{4.53}$$

where the real number q denotes an entropic index that characterizes the degree of non-extensivity. Equation (4.53) demonstrates Shannon entropy when $q \rightarrow 1$ [43]. Tsallis entropy is non-extensive for a statistically dependent system. Its entropy is defined to obey the pseudo additivity rule:

$$S_q(A+B) = S_q(A) + S_q(B) + (1-q) \times S_q(A) \times S_q(B) \tag{4.54}$$

Three different entropies can be defined with regard to different values of q:

- For $q < 1$, the Tsallis entropy becomes a sub-extensive entropy where $S_q(A+B) < S_q(A) + S_q(B)$.
- For $q = 1$, the Tsallis entropy reduces to an standard extensive entropy where $S_q(A+B) = S_q(A) + S_q(B)$.
- For $q > 1$, Tsallis entropy becomes a super-extensive entropy where $S_q(A+B) > S_q(A) + S_q(B)$.

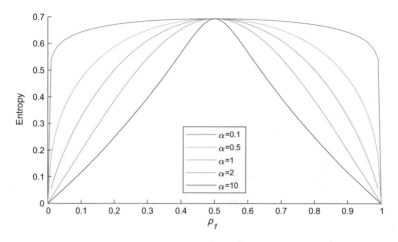

Fig. 4.11 Renyi entropy with various α-values

4.8.3 Renyi Entropy

Renyi entropy [44] of order α is defined as:

$$S_\alpha(X) = \frac{1}{1-\alpha} \log\left(\sum_i P_i^\alpha\right) \tag{4.55}$$

where S_α represents Renyi entropy, with $\alpha \geq 0$ and $\alpha \neq 1$. In some special cases, Renyi entropy will turn to other types of entropy. For instance, $S_0(X)$ is called Hartley entropy, $S_1(X)$ Shannon entropy, and $S_\infty(X)$ min-entropy.

Suppose a binary random variable X with $P = [p_1, p_2]$, where $p_2 = 1 - p_1$. Renyi entropy, with various α-values, is plotted against p_1 in Fig. 4.11. The concaveness and the non-increasing properties against α are obvious from this picture [45].

4.9 Conclusion

This chapter summarized the canonical features for PBD. In addition to the abovementioned feature extraction methods, there are many other novel methods, e.g., fractal dimension, eigenbrain (EB), displacement field, curve-like structure. Readers are encouraged to test such feature extraction methods using images of their own.

References

1. Mazuran M, Tipaldi GD, Spinello L, Burgard W, Stachniss C (2014) A statistical measure for map consistency in SLAM. In: International conference on robotics and automation, Hong Kong, P.R. CHINA IEEE international conference on robotics and automation ICRA. IEEE, pp 3650–3655

2. Dong Z, Ji G (2015) Effect of spider-web-plot in MR brain image classification. Pattern Recogn Lett 62:14–16. https://doi.org/10.1016/j.patrec.2015.04.016

3. Hu H, Li Y, Liu M, Liang W (2014) Classification of defects in steel strip surface based on multiclass support vector machine. Multimed Tools Appl 69(1):199–216. https://doi.org/10.1007/s11042-012-1248-0

4. Ying XH, Hou LL, Hou YB, Kong J, Zha HB (2013) Canonicalized central absolute moment for edge-based color constancy. In: 20th International conference on image processing (ICIP), Melbourne, Austrailia. IEEE, pp 2260–2263

5. Hu M-K (1962) Visual pattern recognition by moment invariants. IRE Trans Inf Theory 8 (2):179–187. https://doi.org/10.1109/TIT.1962.1057692

6. Sun P (2015) Pathological brain detection based on wavelet entropy and Hu moment invariants. Bio-Med Mater Eng 26(s1):1283–1290. https://doi.org/10.2528/PIER13121310

7. Yang J (2017) Pathological brain detection in MRI scanning via Hu moment invariants and machine learning. J Exp Theor Artif Intell 29(2):299–312. https://doi.org/10.1080/0952813X.2015.1132274

8. Zunic J, Hirota K, Dukic D, Aktas MA (2016) On a 3D analogue of the first Hu moment invariant and a family of shape ellipsoidness measures. Mach Vis Appl 27(1):129–144. https://doi.org/10.1007/s00138-015-0730-x

9. Tahmasbi A, Saki F, Shokouhi SB (2011) Classification of benign and malignant masses based on Zernike moments. Comput Biol Med 41(8):726–735. https://doi.org/10.1016/j.compbiomed.2011.06.009

10. Sharma S, Khanna P (2015) Computer-aided diagnosis of malignant mammograms using zernike moments and SVM. J Digit Imaging 28(1):77–90. https://doi.org/10.1007/s10278-014-9719-7

11. Farokhi S, Sheikh UU, Flusser J, Yang B (2015) Near infrared face recognition using Zernike moments and Hermite kernels. Inf Sci 316:234–245. https://doi.org/10.1016/j.ins.2015.04.030

12. Dai XB, Liu TL, Shu HZ, Luo LM (2014) Pseudo-Zernike moment invariants to blur degradation and similarity transformation. Int J Comput Math 91(11):2403–2414. https://doi.org/10.1080/00207160.2013.831083

13. Hu W, Liu HT, Hu C, Wang SG, Chen D, Mo JQ, Liang QH (2013) Vision-based force measurement using pseudo-zernike moment invariants. Measurement 46(10):4293–4305. https://doi.org/10.1016/j.measurement.2013.08.022

14. Shi Z, Liu GX, Du MH (2012) Rotary face recognition based on pseudo-Zernike moment. In: Mao E, Xu LL, Tian W (eds) Emerging computation and information technologies for education, vol 146. Advances in intelligent and soft computing. Springer-Verlag, Berlin, Berlin, pp 641–646

15. Hosny KM (2012) Accurate pseudo Zernike moment invariants for grey-level images. Imaging Sci J 60(4):234–242. https://doi.org/10.1179/1743131x11y.0000000023

16. Gorji HT, Haddadnia J (2015) A novel method for early diagnosis of Alzheimer's disease based on pseudo Zernike moment from structural MRI. Neuroscience 305:361–371. https://doi.org/10.1016/j.neuroscience.2015.08.013

17. Du S (2017) Alzheimer's disease detection by pseudo Zernike moment and linear regression classification. CNS Neurol Disord Drug Targets 16(1):11–15

18. Mokni R, Kherallah M (2016) Palmprint identification using GLCM texture features extraction and SVM classifier. J Inf Assur Secur 11(2):77–86

19. Malegori C, Franzetti L, Guidetti R, Casiraghi E, Rossi R (2016) GLCM, an image analysis technique for early detection of biofilm. J Food Eng 185:48–55. https://doi.org/10.1016/j.jfoodeng.2016.04.001

20. Yousefi Banaem H, Mehri Dehnavi A, Shahnazi M (2015) Ensemble supervised classification method using the regions of interest and grey level co-occurrence matrices features for mammograms data. Iran J Radiol 12(3), Article ID: e11656. https://doi.org/10.5812/iranjradiol.11656

21. Fathima MM, Manimegalai D, Thaiyalnayaki S (2013) Automatic detection of tumor subtype in mammograms based on GLCM and DWT features using SVM. In: International conference on information communication and embedded systems, Chennai, INDIA. IEEE, pp 809–813

22. Zvoleff A (2016) Package "glcm". https://cran.r-project.org/web/packages/glcm/glcm.pdf

23. Haralick RM, Shanmugam K (1973) Textural features for image classification. IEEE Trans Syst Man Cybern SMC-3(6):610–621

24. Pal B (2017) Fourier Transform Ultrasound Spectroscopy for the determination of wave propagation parameters. Ultrasonics 73:140–143. https://doi.org/10.1016/j.ultras.2016.09.008

25. Madhukar BN, Jain S (2016) A duality theorem for the discrete sine transform–IV(DST–IV). In: 3rd international conference on advanced computing and communication systems, Chennai, India, IEEE, pp 206–211

26. Park CS (2016) Two-dimensional discrete cosine transform on sliding windows. Digit Signal Proc 58:20–25. https://doi.org/10.1016/j.dsp.2016.07.011

27. Parot V, Sing-Long C, Lizama C, Tejos C, Uribe S, Irarrazaval P (2012) Application of the fractional Fourier transform to image reconstruction in MRI. Magn Reson Med 68(1):17–29. https://doi.org/10.1002/mrm.23190

28. Li J (2016) Detection of left-sided and right-sided hearing loss via fractional Fourier transform. Entropy 18(5), Article ID: 194. https://doi.org/10.3390/e18050194

29. Liu G (2016) Computer-aided diagnosis of abnormal breasts in mammogram images by weighted-type fractional Fourier transform. Adv Mech Eng 8(2), Article ID: 11. https://doi.org/10.1177/1687814016634243

30. Shih C-C (1995) Fractionalization of Fourier transform. Opt Commun 118 (5–6): 495–498. https://doi.org/10.1016/0030-4018(95)00268-d

31. Santhanam B, McClellan JH (1996) The discrete rotational Fourier transform. IEEE Trans Signal Process 44(4):994–998. https://doi.org/10.1109/78.492554

32. Chen S, Yang J-F, Phillips P (2015) Magnetic resonance brain image classification based on weighted-type fractional Fourier transform and nonparallel support vector machine. Int J Imaging Syst Technol 25(4):317–327. https://doi.org/10.1002/ima.22144

33. Ozaktas HM, Arikan O, Kutay MA, Bozdagt G (1996) Digital computation of the fractional Fourier transform. IEEE Trans Signal Process 44(9):2141–2150. https://doi.org/10.1109/78.536672

34. Namias V (1980) The fractional order Fourier transform and its application to quantum mechanics. IMA J Appl Math 25(3):241–265. https://doi.org/10.1093/imamat/25.3.241

35. Pei S-C, Yeh M-H (1997) Improved discrete fractional Fourier transform. Opt Lett 22 (14):1047–1049. https://doi.org/10.1364/OL.22.001047

36. Dickinson BW, Steiglitz K (1982) Eigenvectors and functions of the discrete Fourier transform. IEEE Trans Acoust Speech Signal Process 30(1):25–31. https://doi.org/10.1109/TASSP.1982.1163843

37. Guida A, Nienow AW, Barigou M (2010) Shannon entropy for local and global description of mixing by Lagrangian particle tracking. Chem Eng Sci 65(10):2865–2883

38. Sun Y (2016) A multilayer perceptron based smart pathological brain detection system by fractional Fourier entropy. J Med Syst 40(7), Article ID: 173. https://doi.org/10.1007/s10916-016-0525-2

39. Cattani C, Rao R (2016) Tea category identification using a novel fractional Fourier entropy and Jaya algorithm. Entropy 8(3), Article ID: 77. https://doi.org/10.3390/e18030077

40. Yang X, Sun P, Dong Z, Liu A, Yuan T-F (2015) Pathological brain detection by a novel image feature—fractional Fourier entropy. Entropy 17(12):8278–8296. https://doi.org/10.3390/e17127877
41. Yang J (2015) Preclinical diagnosis of magnetic resonance (MR) brain images via discrete wavelet packet transform with Tsallis entropy and generalized eigenvalue proximal support vector machine (GEPSVM). Entropy 17(4):1795–1813. https://doi.org/10.3390/e17041795
42. Tsallis C (2009) Nonadditive entropy: the concept and its use. Eur Phys J A 40(3):257–266. https://doi.org/10.1140/epja/i2009-10799-0
43. Wu LN (2008) Pattern recognition via PCNN and Tsallis entropy. Sensors 8(11):7518–7529. https://doi.org/10.3390/s8117518
44. Mora T, Walczak AM (2016) Renyi entropy, abundance distribution, and the equivalence of ensembles. Phys Rev E 93(5), Article ID: 052418. https://doi.org/10.1103/physreve.93.052418
45. Han L (2018) Identification of Alcoholism based on wavelet Renyi entropy and three-segment encoded Jaya algorithm. Complexity, Article ID: 3198184

Chapter 5
Multi-scale and Multi-resolution Features for Structural Magnetic Resonance Imaging

This chapter is a natural follow on from Chap. 4, focusing on multiscale and multiresolution features. First, the development of signal processing from Fourier transform to short-time Fourier transform to wavelet analysis, is presented. The advantages and disadvantages of the three techniques are analyzed. Next, the question of why wavelet transform is the most popular feature extraction method is answered, by comparison between fingerprints and brain gyri. An explanation of the continuous wavelet transform is given with a Koch curve example. The discrete wavelet transform is deduced by replacing a continuous variable with a discrete variable. The relationship between decomposition and reconstruction is explained. In addition, the effect of low-pass filters and high-pass filters on the wavelet transform is estimated. Four Matlab commands: "dwt," "idwt," "wavedec," and "waverec" are introduced and analyzed. Further, we show how to extend a 1D wavelet transform to 2D and 3D, analyzing their Matlab commands. A three-level 3D discrete wavelet transform of the human brain is also given.

5.1 Wavelet Transform

5.1.1 Development of Signal Processing

The most conventional tool for signal analysis is the Fourier transform (FT), which breaks down a time domain signal into constituent sinusoids of different frequencies, thus, transforming the signal from time domain to frequency domain.

However, FT has a serious drawback. It results in the loss of time information from the signal. For example, an analyst cannot tell when a particular event took place by looking at a Fourier spectrum. Thus, classification accuracy will decrease as time information is lost.

© Springer Nature Singapore Pte Ltd. 2018
S.-H. Wang et al., *Pathological Brain Detection*, Brain Informatics and Health,
https://doi.org/10.1007/978-981-10-4026-9_5

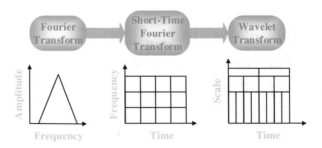

Fig. 5.1 Development of signal processing

Gabor adapted the FT to analyze only a small section of the signal at a time. The technique is called windowing or short-time Fourier transform (STFT) [1]. It adds a window of a particular shape to the signal. A STFT can be regarded as a compromise between the time information and frequency information [2]. It provides some information about both the time domain and frequency domain. However, the precision of the information is limited by the size of the window [3].

Figure 5.1 shows that the wavelet transform (WT) represents the next logical step: a windowing technique with variable size. Thus, it preserves both the time and frequency information of the signal.

The WT adopts "scale" instead of traditional "frequency," namely, it does not produce a time–frequency view but a time–scale view of the signal. The time–scale view is a different way to view data, but is more natural and powerful.

5.1.2 Potential Application to Pathological Brain Detection

The WT is successfully applied in fingerprint identification [4, 5], the sensors of which are shown in Fig. 5.2. Here the pictures show two fingerprint sensors on the back of a cell phone and on a laptop.

The similarities between fingerprints and the brain gyri (Fig. 5.3) motivated scholars to apply the WT to brain images. The multiscale analysis of wavelet help to find the texture pattern of the brain images. The prominent achievements of applying wavelet for brain image analysis are described in Chap. 10.

When using the discrete wavelet transform (DWT) for pathological brain classification, it is usually combined with other statistical techniques, e.g., wavelet entropy, wavelet energy, wavelet variance [6], wavelet energy entropy [7], etc.

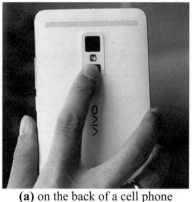

(a) on the back of a cell phone

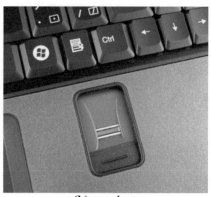

(b) on a laptop

Fig. 5.2 Applications of fingerprint identification sensors

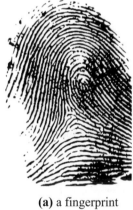

(a) a fingerprint

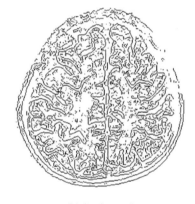

(b) brain gyri

Fig. 5.3 Similarities between fingerprints and the brain gyri

5.2 Continuous Wavelet Transform and Discrete Wavelet Transform

5.2.1 Mathematical Analysis of a Continuous Wavelet Transform

Suppose $I(t)$ is a square-integrable function, then the continuous wavelet transform (CWT) [8] of $x(t)$ relative to a given wavelet $\psi(t)$ is defined as:

Table 5.1 The "cwt"
command

coefs = cwt(x, scales, wname)
Input x: input signal scales: one-dimensional vector with positive elements wname: wavelet name
Output coefs: continuous wavelet transform coefficients

$$W_\psi(a,b) = \int\limits_{-\infty}^{\infty} I(t)\psi_{a,b}(t)\,\mathrm{d}t \qquad (5.1)$$

where

$$\psi_{a,b}(t) = \frac{1}{\sqrt{a}}\psi\left(\frac{t-a}{b}\right) \qquad (5.2)$$

Here, the wavelet $\psi_{a,b}(t)$ is calculated from the mother wavelet $\psi(t)$ by translation and dilation [9]: a is the dilation factor and b is the translation parameter (both real, positive numbers) [10].

Table 5.1 details the "cwt" Matlab command.

5.2.2   Koch Curve Example of the Continuous Wavelet Transform

In this section, we used the von Koch curve as an example, which is shown in Fig. 5.4. The CWT is shown in Fig. 5.5. Here the decomposition scale of the CWT is from 1 to 64.

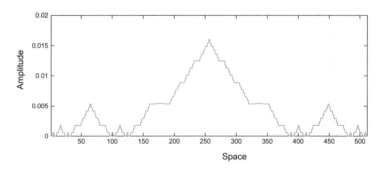

Fig. 5.4 The von Koch curve

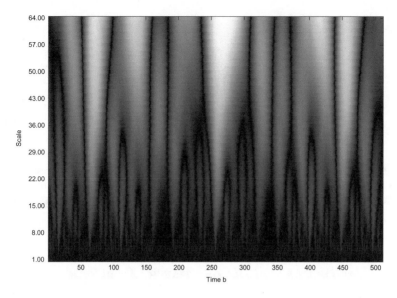

Fig. 5.5 The CWT of the von Koch curve

5.2.3   Discrete Wavelet Transform

The DWT discretized Eq. (5.1) using following settings:

$$a = 2^{-j} \tag{5.3}$$

$$b = k \times 2^{-j} \tag{5.4}$$

Suppose a low-pass filter (LPF) g and a high-pass filter (HPF) h are created, we have:

$$c_a(j,k) = \left(\sum_n I(n) g_j^* \left(n - 2^j k \right) \right) \downarrow 2 \tag{5.5}$$

$$c_d(j,k) = \left(\sum_n I(n) h_j^* \left(n - 2^j k \right) \right) \downarrow 2 \tag{5.6}$$

where c_a and c_d are approximation coefficients and detail coefficients, respectively [11], and $\downarrow$ is defined as the downsampling operator:

$$(I \downarrow k)[n] = I[kn] \tag{5.7}$$

where n is the discrete version of time t.

Fig. 5.6 Three-level 1D
DWT

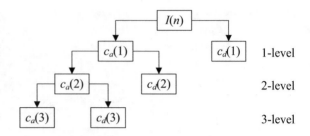

The above decomposition process can be iterated with successive approxima-
tions being decomposed in turn, so that one signal is broken down into various
levels of resolution. Figure 5.6 shows the three-level 1D DWT procedure. Here the
j in $c_a(j)$ and $c_d(j)$ represents the decomposition level [12].

5.2.4 One-Dimensional Discrete Wavelet Transform Commands

Four important Matlab commands are introduced. The "dwt" and "idwt" commands
can be used to decompose and reconstruct the single-level 1D DWT, respectively.
Tables 5.2 and 5.3 detail these two commands.

The two other commands "wavedec" and "waverec" can perform the multilevel
1D DWT. Their parameters are shown in Tables 5.4 and 5.5.

Table 5.2 The "dwt"
command

[cA, cD] = dwt (X, wname)
Input X: input vector wname: wavelet name
Output cA: approximation coefficients cD: detail coefficients

Table 5.3 The "idwt"
command

X = idwt (cA, cD, wname)
Input cA: approximation coefficients cD: detail coefficients wname: wavelet name
Output X: reconstructed signal

Table 5.4 The "wavedec" command

[C, L] = wavedec (X, N, wname)
Input X: input vector N: decomposition level wname: wavelet name
Output C: stores the coefficients of each subband L: stores the lengths of each subband

Table 5.5 The "waverec" command

X = waverec(C, L, wname)
Input C: stores the coefficients of each subband L: stores the lengths of each subband wname: wavelet name
Output X: reconstructed signal

5.3   From One-Dimensional to Two-Dimensional to Three-Dimensional

Since we understand the 1D DWT, we shall extend it to the 2D and 3D DWT in this section.

5.3.1   Two-Dimensional Discrete Wavelet Transform

When I is extended to become a 2D brain image, the 1D DWT is applied to row and column directions separately [13]. Figure 5.7 shows the diagram of a three-level 2D DWT.

The horizontal c_h sub-band is obtained by passing image I through an HPF along the x-axis [14] and an LPF along the y-axis:

$$c_h(x, y) = \sum_{m,n} I(m, n) \times h(2x - m) \times g(2y - n) \qquad (5.8)$$

The vertical c_v sub-band is obtained by passing the image s through an LPF along the x-axis and an HPF along the y-axis [15]:

$$c_v(x, y) = \sum_{m,n} I(m, n) \times g(2x - m) \times h(2y - n) \qquad (5.9)$$

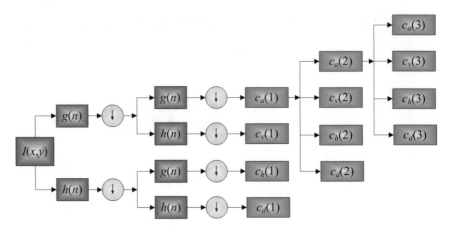

Fig. 5.7 Diagram of the three-level 2D DWT

The approximation sub-band c_a is obtained by passing through LPFs along both axes:

$$c_a(x, y) = \sum_{m,n} I(m, n) \times g(2x - m) \times g(2y - n) \qquad (5.10)$$

The diagonal sub-band c_d is obtained by passing through HPFs along both axes:

$$c_d(x, y) = \sum_{m,n} I(m, n) \times h(2x - m) \times h(2y - n) \qquad (5.11)$$

Figure 5.8 shows the 2D DWT of a multiple sclerosis brain image. A pseudo colormap has been added to improve visual quality. We find that more detailed sub-bands are generated with an increase of decomposition level [16].

5.3.2 Two-Dimensional Discrete Wavelet Transform Commands

This section gives the Matlab commands for the 2D DWT. Similar to the contents of Sect. 5.2.4, four key commands are introduced:

- "dwt2" and "idwt2" perform single-level 2D DWT decomposition and reconstruction, respectively (Tables 5.6 and 5.7).
- "wavedec2" and "waverec2" perform multilevel 2D DWT decomposition and reconstruction, respectively (Tables 5.8 and 5.9).

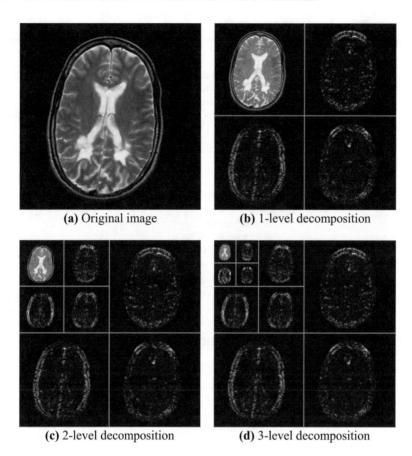

(a) Original image   (b) 1-level decomposition

(c) 2-level decomposition   (d) 3-level decomposition

Fig. 5.8 Illustration of the 2D DWT over a multiple sclerosis brain image

Table 5.6 The "dwt2" command	**[cA, cH, cV, cD] = dwt2(X, wname)**
	Input X: input matrix wname: wavelet name
	Output cA: approximation coefficients cH: horizontal coefficients cV: vertical coefficients cD: diagonal coefficients

Table 5.7 The "idwt2" command

X = idwt2(cA, cH, cV, cD, wname)
Input
cA: approximation coefficients
cH: horizontal coefficients
cV: vertical coefficients
cD: diagonal coefficients
wname: wavelet name
Output
X: reconstructed matrix

Table 5.8 The "wavedec2" command

[C,S] = wavedec2(X, N, wname)
Input
X: input matrix
N: decomposition level
wname: wavelet name
Output
C: stores the coefficients of each subband
S: stores the sizes of each subband

Table 5.9 The "waverec2" command

X = waverec2(C, S, wname)
Input
C: stores the coefficients of each subband
S: stores the sizes of each subband
wname: wavelet name
Output
X: reconstructed matrix

5.4   Three-Dimensional Discrete Wavelet Transform

5.4.1   Decomposition Diagram

Using similar technique used for 2D, we can extend to it to the situation in which I is a 3D volumetric brain image. In simple words, we implement the 3D DWT by applying the 1D DWT to row, column, and slice directions, separately [17]. Figure 5.9 shows a diagram for the 3D DWT.

Note that in this 3D situation [18], we did not use a, h, v, and d to represent different coefficient sub-bands. Instead, we used LLL, LLH, LHL, LHH, HLL, HLH, HHL, and HHH to represent the eight sub-bands in the 3D DWT [19]. Here L means the result after an LPF, and H means the result after an HPF.

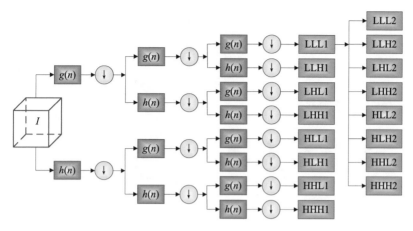

Fig. 5.9 Diagram of a 2-level 3D DWT

5.4.2   Illustration of the Three-Dimensional Discrete Wavelet Transform

Figure 5.10 shows the 1-level 3D DWT result for a cube. Figure 5.11 shows a 3D image of the head. Figures 5.12, 5.13, and 5.14 show respectively the corresponding 1-level, 2-level, and 3-level 3D DWT decomposition results for the head.

There are four corresponding Matlab commands related to the 3D DWT:

- "dwt3" and "idwt3" perform single-level 3D DWT decomposition and reconstruction, respectively.
- "wavedec3" and "waverec3" perform multilevel 3D DWT decomposition and reconstruction, respectively.

Here we have not shown details of the four commands due to their similarity with the 1D DWT and the 2D DWT.

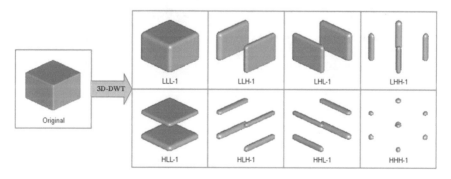

Fig. 5.10 The 1-level 3D DWT of a cube

Fig. 5.11 A 3D image of the head

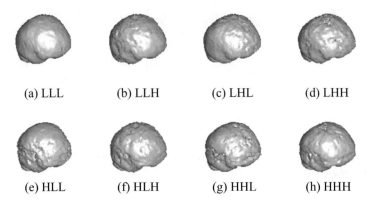

(a) LLL	(b) LLH	(c) LHL	(d) LHH
(e) HLL	(f) HLH	(g) HHL	(h) HHH

Fig. 5.12 The 1-level 3D DWT for a 3D image of the head

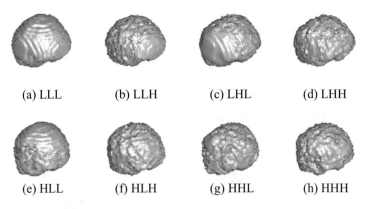

(a) LLL	(b) LLH	(c) LHL	(d) LHH
(e) HLL	(f) HLH	(g) HHL	(h) HHH

Fig. 5.13 The 2-level 3D DWT for a 3D image of the head

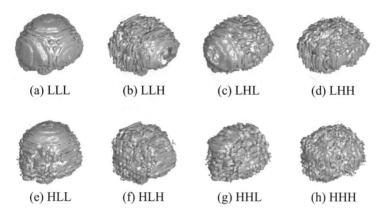

(a) LLL	(b) LLH	(c) LHL	(d) LHH
(e) HLL	(f) HLH	(g) HHL	(h) HHH

Fig. 5.14 The 3-level 3D DWT for a 3D image of the head

5.5   Conclusion

This chapter gives a preliminary overview of wavelet transform and explains why wavelets can be applied to PBD to some degree. Readers are encouraged to use the Matlab commands in this chapter in order to test their performance.

References

1. Garrido M (2016) The feedforward short-time fourier transform. IEEE Trans Circuits Syst II Express Briefs 63(9):868–872. https://doi.org/10.1109/tcsii.2016.2534838
2. Lisicki M, D'Ostilio K, Nonis R, Schoenen J, Magis D (2016) Habituation in sub-components of visual evoked potentials: a short-time fourier transform analysis in healthy and migraine subjects. Cephalalgia 36:55
3. Balazs P, Bayer D, Jaillet F, Sondergaard P (2016) The pole behavior of the phase derivative of the short-time fourier transform. Appl Comput Harmonic Anal 40(3):610–621. https://doi.org/10.1016/j.acha.2015.10.001
4. Shinde MK, Annadate SA (2015) Analysis of fingerprint image for gender classification or identification using wavelet transform and singular value decomposition. In: 1st international conference on computing communication control and automation Iccubea, Pune, India, IEEE, pp 650–654. https://doi.org/10.1109/iccubea.2015.133
5. Khalil MS (2015) Reference point detection for camera-based fingerprint image based on wavelet transformation. Biomed Eng Online 14:23, Article ID: 40. https://doi.org/10.1186/s12938-015-0029-1
6. Vernotte F, Lenczner M, Bourgeois PY, Rubiola E (2016) The parabolic variance (PVAR): a wavelet variance based on the least-square fit. IEEE Trans Ultrason Ferroelectr Freq Control 63(4):611–623. https://doi.org/10.1109/tuffc.2015.2499325
7. Chen Y, Zhang Y, Lu H (2016) Wavelet energy entropy and linear regression classifier for detecting abnormal breasts. Multimedia Tools Appl. https://doi.org/10.1007/s11042-016-4161-0

8. Pandey JN, Jha NK, Singh OP (2016) The continuous wavelet transform in n-dimensions. Int J Wavelets Multiresolut Inf Process 14(5), Article ID: 1650037. https://doi.org/10.1142/s0219691316500375
9. Fang L, Wu L (2015) A novel demodulation system based on continuous wavelet transform. Math Probl Eng, Article ID: 513849. https://doi.org/10.1155/2015/513849
10. Gholizad A, Safari H (2016) Two-dimensional continuous wavelet transform method for multidamage detection of space structures. J Perform Constr Facil 30(6):14, Article ID: 04016064. https://doi.org/10.1061/(asce)cf.1943-5509.0000924
11. Huo Y (2010) Feature extraction of brain MRI by stationary wavelet transform and its applications. J Biol Syst 18(S):115–132
12. Han L (2018) Identification of alcoholism based on wavelet Renyi entropy and three-segment encoded Jaya algorithm. Complexity 2018, Article ID: 3198184
13. Hong GS, Kim BG, Hwang YS, Kwon KK (2016) Fast multi-feature pedestrian detection algorithm based on histogram of oriented gradient using discrete wavelet transform. Multimedia Tools Appl 75(23):15229–15245. https://doi.org/10.1007/s11042-015-2455-2
14. Gorriz JM, Ramírez J (2016) Wavelet entropy and directed acyclic graph support vector machine for detection of patients with unilateral hearing loss in MRI scanning. Front Comput Neurosci 10, Article ID: 160. https://doi.org/10.3389/fncom.2016.00100
15. Al-Azawi S (2018) Low-power, low-area multi-level 2-D discrete wavelet transform architecture. Circuits Syst Sign Process 37(1):444–458. https://doi.org/10.1007/s00034-017-0553-2
16. Chabchoub S, Mansouri S, Ben Salah R (2016) Impedance cardiography signal denoising using discrete wavelet transform. Australas Phys Eng Sci Med 39(3):655–663. https://doi.org/10.1007/s13246-016-0460-z
17. Ghasemzadeh A, Demirel H (2018) 3D discrete wavelet transform-based feature extraction for hyperspectral face recognition. IET Biometrics 7(1):49–55. https://doi.org/10.1049/iet-bmt.2017.0082
18. Chen Y, Lee E (2015) 3D-DWT improves prediction of AD and MCI. In: Ding J (ed) Advances in computer science research, vol 3. ACSR-advances in computer science research. Atlantis Press, Paris, pp 60–63
19. Phillips P, Dong Z, Ji G, Yang J (2015) Detection of alzheimer's disease and mild cognitive impairment based on structural volumetric MR images using 3D-DWT and WTA-KSVM trained by PSOTVAC. Biomed Sign Process Control 21:58–73. https://doi.org/10.1016/j.bspc.2015.05.014

Chapter 6
Wavelet Families and Variants

In this chapter, four important wavelet families are discussed: the Daubechies wavelet family, the Coiflet wavelet family, the Morlet wavelet family, and the biorthogonal wavelet family. The wavelet display function and the "waveinfo" command are introduced so that the detailed curve shape of scaling and wavelet functions, for both decomposition and reconstruction, can be viewed in arbitrary accuracy. Several popular wavelet transform variants are presented. The ε-decimated wavelet transform chooses either odd or even index randomly. The stationary wavelet transform (SWT) calculates all the ε-decimated discrete wavelet transforms (DWTs) and provides an average. A wavelet packet transform (WPT) passes all coefficients (both approximation and detail) through
quadrature mirror filters to create a full binary tree. The dual-tree complex wavelet transform (DTCWT) is carried out by two separate two-channel filter banks, to enhance the directional selectivity compared to the standard DWT. In addition, the scaling and wavelet filters in the DTCWT cannot be selected arbitrarily. Finally, the "wavelet design and analysis" app in the wavelet toolbox found in the Matlab software is illustrated.

6.1 Wavelet Families

In this section, we shall introduce several widely used wavelet families [1].

6.1.1 Daubechies Wavelets

First is the Daubechies family of wavelets (abbreviated as db). They are orthogonal wavelets, characterized by a maximal number of vanishing moments for a given support. With each wavelet, there is a corresponding scaling function generating an

© Springer Nature Singapore Pte Ltd. 2018
S.-H. Wang et al., *Pathological Brain Detection*, Brain Informatics and Health,
https://doi.org/10.1007/978-981-10-4026-9_6

orthogonal multiresolution analysis. Note that db1 is the same as the Haar wavelet. Besides this, the symlet wavelets are a series of modified versions of Daubechies wavelets with increased symmetry. Figures 6.1 and 6.2 show the scaling functions and wavelet functions, respectively, of db1 to db9.

6.1.2 Coiflet Wavelets

Coiflets are another family of wavelets (abbreviated as coif). They are near symmetric [2]. Their scaling function has ($N/3-1$) vanishing moments, and the wavelet function has $N/3$ vanishing moments [3]. Figures 6.3 and 6.4 show the scaling functions and wavelet functions, respectively, of the Coiflet family.

6.1.3 Morlet Wavelets

Morlet wavelets, are a wavelet family composed of a complex exponential multiplied by a Gaussian window [4]. The complex exponential can be regarded as the carrier, while the Gaussian window can be regarded as the envelope [5]. Morlet wavelets are related to human perception, e.g., vision and hearing. Figure 6.5 shows the wavelet function of a real-valued Morlet, which does not have a scaling function. Figure 6.6 shows the wavelet function of a complex-valued Morlet (also called a Gabor wavelet [6]).

6.1.4 Biorthogonal Wavelets

A biorthogonal wavelet (abbreviated as bior) has two scaling functions and two wavelet functions [7, 8]. One scaling/wavelet function is for decomposition, the other is for reconstruction. Figures 6.7, 6.8, and 6.9 give all the functions of bior2.2, bior3.3, and bior4.4, respectively.

Note that the "wfilters" command can compute the four filters associated with orthogonal or biorthogonal wavelets. The input and output parameters of "wfilters" are given in Table 6.1.

6.1.5 Matlab Commands

There are some other important wavelet families, such as Meyer wavelets, Mexican hat wavelets, Shannon wavelets [9], B-spline wavelets, reverse biorthogonal wavelets (abbreviated as rbio) [10], etc. Readers can draw these wavelets using the

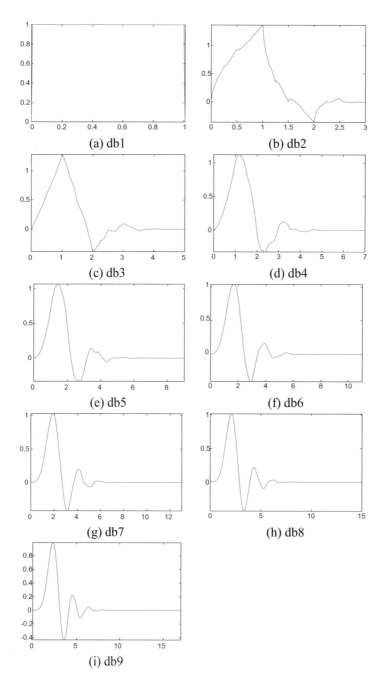

Fig. 6.1 Scaling functions of the Daubechies family of wavelets (*x* axis is time and *y* axis is amplitude)

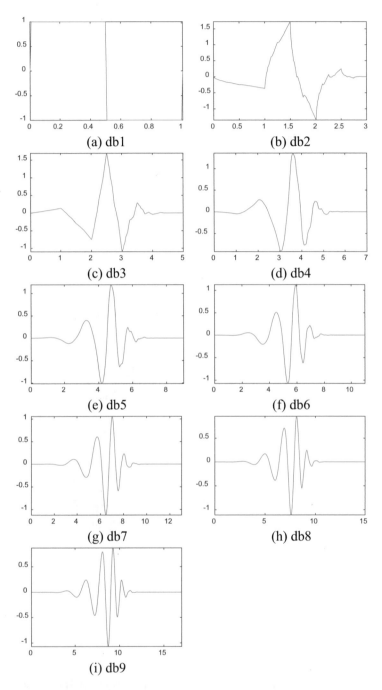

Fig. 6.2 Wavelet functions of the Daubechies family of wavelets (*x* axis is time and *y* axis is amplitude)

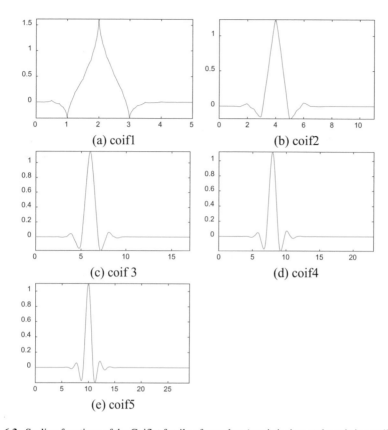

Fig. 6.3 Scaling functions of the Coiflet family of wavelets (*x* axis is time and *y* axis is amplitude)

"wavelet display" functions in Matlab. For example, Fig. 6.10 gives the wavelet display related to the rbio3.3 wavelet.

The Matlab command "waveinfo" can provide information on all wavelets, which are held within the Matlab software. For example, we can obtain the basic information about the Haar wavelet and the Shannon wavelet using the following two commands:

- The "waveinfo('haar')" command returns the information given in Table 6.2.
- The "waveinfo('shan')" command returns the information given Table 6.3.

Another important command is "wavemngr," which is a type of wavelet manger which allows the user to add, delete, restore, or read wavelets.

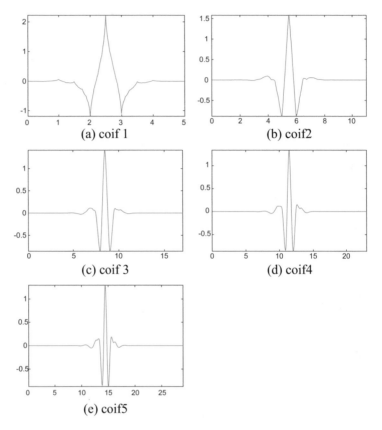

Fig. 6.4 Wavelet functions of the Coiflet family of wavelets (*x* axis is time and *y* axis is amplitude)

Fig. 6.5 Wavelet function of a real-valued Morlet (*x* axis is time or space and *y* axis is amplitude)

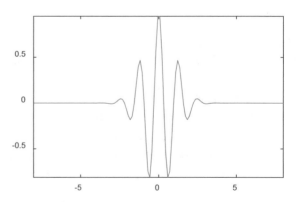

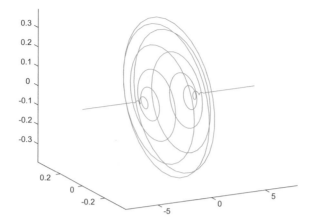

Fig. 6.6 Wavelet function of a complex-valued Morlet

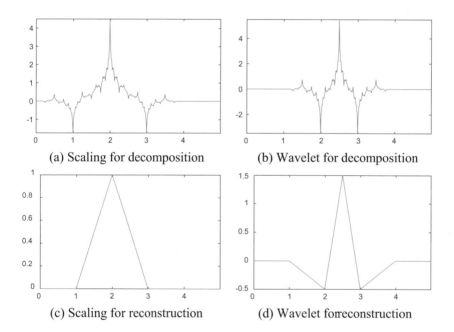

(a) Scaling for decomposition

(b) Wavelet for decomposition

(c) Scaling for reconstruction

(d) Wavelet forreconstruction

Fig. 6.7 Functions of bior2.2

6.2 ε-Decimated Discrete Wavelet Transform

The DWT has proven its success in various academic and industrial fields. Nevertheless, it lacks translation invariance and directional selectivity. Scholars have proposed many variants of the DWT.

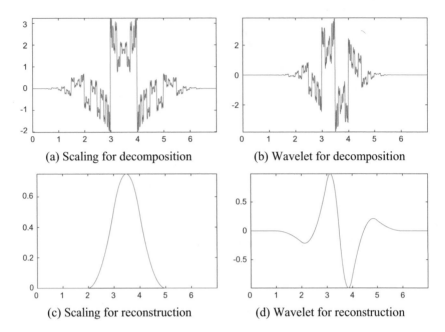

(a) Scaling for decomposition   (b) Wavelet for decomposition

(c) Scaling for reconstruction   (d) Wavelet for reconstruction

Fig. 6.8 Functions of bior3.3

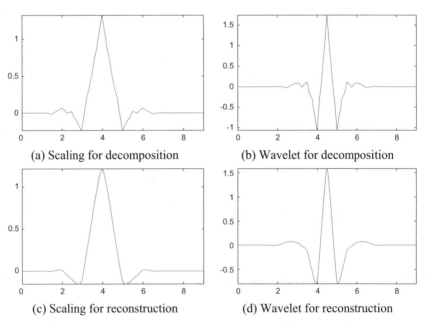

(a) Scaling for decomposition   (b) Wavelet for decomposition

(c) Scaling for reconstruction   (d) Wavelet for reconstruction

Fig. 6.9 Functions of bior4.4

Table 6.1   The "wfilters" command

[LD, HD, LR, HR] = wfilters(wname)
Input wname: wavelet name
Output LD: the decomposition low-pass filter HD: the decomposition high-pass filter LR: the reconstruction low-pass filter HR: the reconstruction high-pass filter

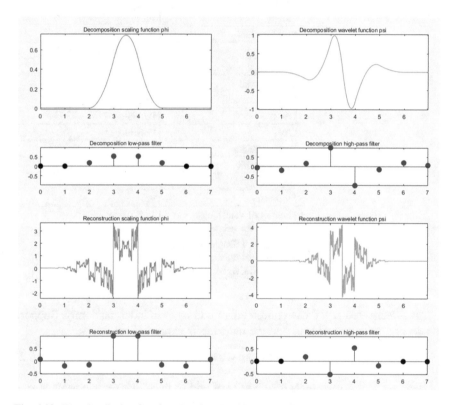

Fig. 6.10   Wavelet display function showing the rbio3.3 wavelet

Suppose I denotes a given magnetic resonance (MR) image, and T the translation operator, then we have:

$$\mathrm{DWT}(T(I)) \neq T(\mathrm{DWT}(I)) \tag{6.1}$$

This is called the "translation invariance" property, which means that the DWT result may change sharply even when the original image was only slightly translated. The reason lies in the decimation method (even-indexed) used in the DWT.

Table 6.2 Information returned using the "waveinfo ('haar')" command

Command: **waveinfo('haar')**	
Result: Information on Haar wavelet	
Haar wavelet	
General characteristics: compactly supported wavelet, the oldest and the simplest wavelet	
Scaling function phi = 1 on [0 1] and 0 otherwise Wavelet function psi = 1 on [0 0.5), = −1 on [0.5 1] and 0 otherwise	
Family	Haar
Short name	Haar
Examples	Haar is the same as db1
Orthogonal	Yes
Biorthogonal	Yes
Compact support	Yes
DWT	Possible
CWT	Possible
Support width	1
Filters length	2
Regularity	Haar is not continuous
Symmetry	yes
Number of vanishing moments for psi	1
Reference: I. Daubechies, Ten lectures on wavelets, CBMS, SIAM, 61, 1994, 194–202	

An ε-decimated DWT can choose either odd or even index randomly. Suppose the decomposition level is J, and the indexing is expressed as:

$$\varepsilon = \varepsilon_1\varepsilon_2...\varepsilon_j...\varepsilon_J \qquad (6.2)$$

Here $\varepsilon_j= 1$ or 0 represents the choices of odd or even indexed elements at step j. A graphical example of $\varepsilon = 0110$ is shown in Fig. 6.11.

6.3　Stationary Wavelet Transform

The SWT calculates all the ε-decimated DWTs for a given signal at one time. More precisely, for level 1, the SWT can be obtained by convolving the signal with the appropriate filters, as in the DWT, but without downsampling [11]. Then the coefficients of the approximation and detail at level 1 are the same as the signal length.

Table 6.3 Information returned using the "waveinfo ('shan')" command

Command:
waveinfo('shan')
Result:
Information on complex Shannon wavelet
Complex Shannon wavelet
Definition: a complex Shannon wavelet is shan(x) = Fb^(0.5)*sinc(Fb*x)*exp(2*i*pi*Fc*x) depending on two parameters: Fb is a bandwidth parameter Fc is a wavelet center frequency
The condition Fc > Fb/2 is sufficient to ensure that zero is not in the frequency support interval

Family	Complex Shannon
Short name	Shan
Wavelet name	Shan"Fb"-"Fc"
Orthogonal	No
Biorthogonal	No
Compact support	No
DWT	No
Complex CWT	Possible
Support width	Infinite

Reference: A. Teolis, Computational signal processing with wavelets, Birkhauser, 1998, 62

Fig. 6.11 Illustration of an ε-decimated DWT with ε = 0110

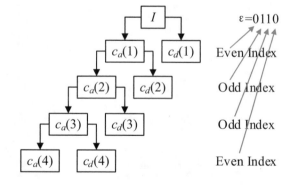

$ε=0110$

Even Index

Odd Index

Odd Index

Even Index

6.3.1 Illustration of the Stationary Wavelet Transform

Figure 6.12 shows SWT results. We can observe that the size of each sub-band is the same as original image. The reason for this is that we have removed the undersampling procedure in the DWT. Note that the SWT is also called the un-decimated wavelet transform (UWT) [12].

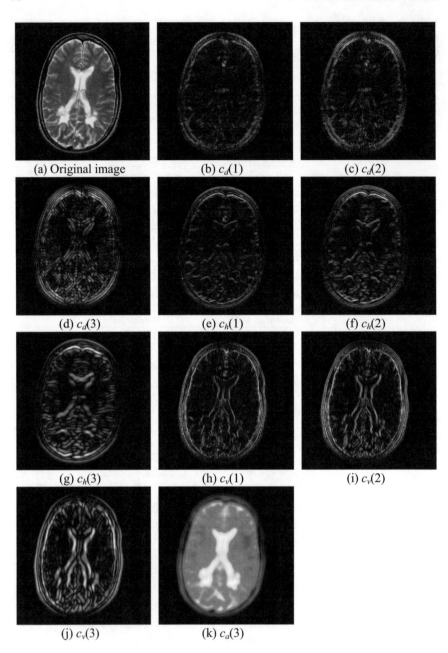

(a) Original image   (b) $c_d(1)$ (c) $c_d(2)$

(d) $c_d(3)$ (e) $c_h(1)$ (f) $c_h(2)$

(g) $c_h(3)$ (h) $c_v(1)$ (i) $c_v(2)$

(j) $c_v(3)$ (k) $c_a(3)$

Fig. 6.12 SWT results (hot colormap is added)

6.3.2 *Matlab Solution*

The Matlab commands "swt" and "iswt" can perform the SWT and inverse SWT— their details are given in Tables 6.4 and 6.5, respectively.

Similarly, "swt2" and "iswt2" can perform 2D SWT decomposition and reconstruction, respectively. Tables 6.6 and 6.7 list their input and output arguments, respectively.

Table 6.4 The "swt" command

SWC = swt(X, N, wname)
Input X: input signal N: decomposition level wname: wavelet name
Output SWC: stationary wavelet coefficients

Table 6.5 The "iswt" command

X = iswt(SWC, wname)
Input SWC: stationary wavelet coefficients wname: wavelet name
Output X: reconstructed signal

Table 6.6 The "swt2" command

SWC = swt2(X, N, wname)
Input X: input matrix N: decomposition level wname: wavelet name
Output SWC: stationary wavelet coefficients

Table 6.7 The "iswt2" command

X = iswt2(SWC, wname)
Input SWC: stationary wavelet coefficients wname: wavelet name
Output X: reconstructed matrix

6.4   Wavelet Packet Transform

The DWT calculates each level by passing only the previous approximation coefficients to quadrature mirror filters (QMFs) [13]. Nevertheless, the WPT [14] passes all coefficients (both approximation and detail) through QMFs to create a full binary tree [15].

6.4.1   Illustration of the Wavelet Packet Transform

Using the same original image in Sect. 5.3.1 we compare the DWT (2-level and 3-level decomposition) with the SWT associated with the same decomposition levels. The results are shown in Fig. 6.13.

6.4.2   Matlab Solution

The decomposition and reconstruction of the 1D WPT can be performed using the "wpdec" and "wprec" commands, respectively. Tables 6.8 and 6.9 show the details of these commands.

Similarly, the decomposition and reconstruction of the 2D WPT can be carried out using the "wpdec2" and "wprec2" commands, the details of which are shown in Tables 6.10 and 6.11, respectively.

6.5   Dual-Tree Complex Wavelet Transform

The standard DWT only has horizontal and vertical directional selectivity, as shown in Fig. 6.14. Here the c_h and c_v have well-defined vertical and horizontal orientations. Nevertheless, c_d mixes directions, that is, −45 and +45 degrees, together, stemming from the use of real-valued filters in the DWT. This mixing severely impedes the direction check [16].

6.5.1   Directional Selectivity

The DTCWT was carried out by two separate two-channel filter banks [17]. Note that the scaling and wavelet filters in the dual-tree cannot be selected arbitrarily. In one tree, the wavelet and scaling filters should produce a wavelet and scaling function, which are approximate Hilbert transforms of those generated by another tree [18].

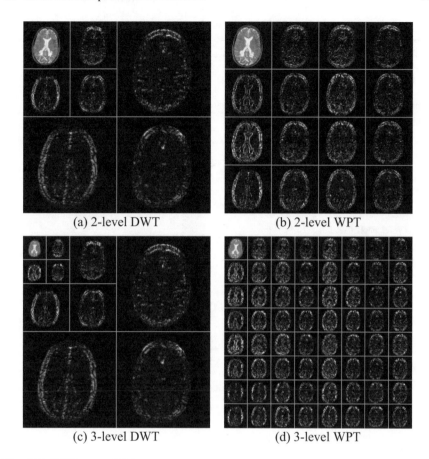

(a) 2-level DWT   (b) 2-level WPT

(c) 3-level DWT   (d) 3-level WPT

Fig. 6.13 DWT versus WPT

Table 6.8 The "wpdec" command

T = wpdec(X, N, wname)
Input X: input signal N: decomposition level wname: wavelet name
Output T: wavelet packet tree

Table 6.9 The "wprec" command

X = wprec(T)
Input T: wavelet packet tree
Output X: reconstructed signal

Table 6.10 The "wpdec2" command

T = wpdec2(X, N, wname)
Input
X: input matrix
N: decomposition level
wname: wavelet name
Output
T: wavelet packet tree

Table 6.11 The "wprec2" command

X = wprec2(T)
Input
T: wavelet packet tree
Output
X: reconstructed matrix

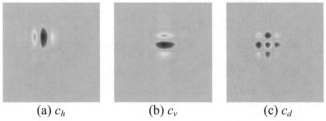

(a) c_h (b) c_v (c) c_d

Fig. 6.14 Directional selectivity of the DWT

In this way, the wavelets generated from both trees, and the complex-valued scaling function, are approximately analytic [19]. At each scale of a 2D DTCWT, six directionally selective sub-bands ($\pm 15°$, $\pm 45°$, $\pm 75°$), for both real (R) and imaginary (I) parts, are produced (Figs. 6.15 and 6.16).

6.5.2 Matlab Solution

Table 6.12 shows that the decomposition of a 1D DTCWT can be performed by the "dddtree" command. Table 6.13 shows that the reconstruction of a 1D DTCWT can be performed by the "idddtree" command. For the 2D situation, the commands are upgraded to "dddtree2" and "idddtree2," respectively.

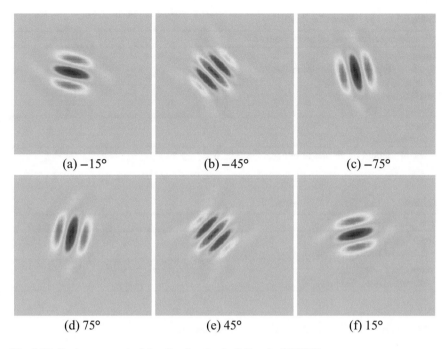

Fig. 6.15 Real component of the directional selectivity of a DTCWT

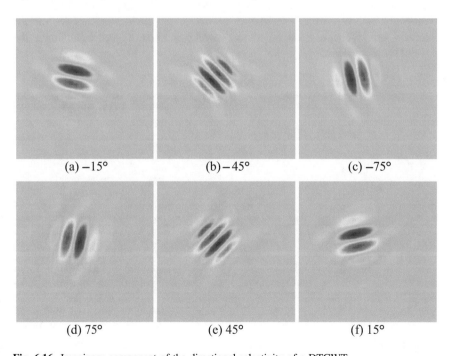

Fig. 6.16 Imaginary component of the directional selectivity of a DTCWT

Table 6.12 The "dddtree" command

wt = dddtree(typetree, x, level, fname)
Input
typetree[a]: type of wavelet decomposition
x: input signal
level: decomposition level
fname: filter name
Output
wt: wavelet transform

([a]"cplxdt" should be chosen to perform the DTCWT)

Table 6.13 The "idddtree" command

xrec = idddtree(wt)
Input
wt: wavelet transform
Output
xrec: reconstructed signal

6.6 Wavelet Design and Analysis App

Figure 6.17 shows the "Wavelet Design and Analysis" app, embedded in the "Wavelet Toolbox," found in Matlab software. It provides access to various graphical user interfaces (GUIs) in the wavelet toolbox. Figure 6.18 shows the wavelet toolbox menu.

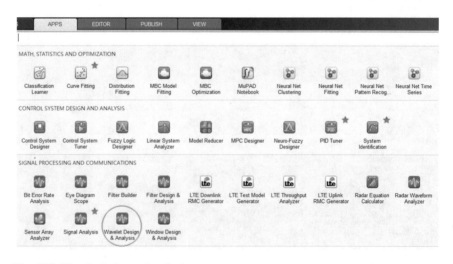

Fig. 6.17 Wavelet design and analysis app

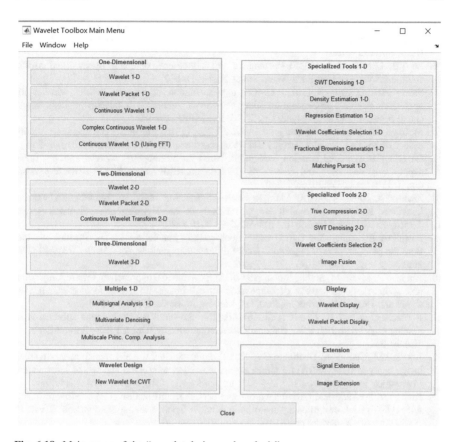

Fig. 6.18 Main menu of the "wavelet design and analysis" app

6.7   Conclusion

This chapter discussed the common wavelet families and variants of the DWT. Readers should note that there are several other excellent wavelet variants: the exponential wavelet transform, the curvelet transform, the contourlet transform, the noiselet transform, etc.

References

1. Bajaj N, Kashyap R (2012) Extension of wavelet family in fractional fourier domain. In: 1st international conference on emerging technology trends in electronics, communication and networking, Surat, India. IEEE, pp 1–4
2. Li LY, Shi KL (2016) Research and realization of transient disturbance detection algorithm based coiflet wavelets and FPGA. Int J Future Gener Commun Network 9(2):133–142

3. Narkhedkar SG, Patel PK (2014) Recipe of speech compression using coiflet wavelet. In: International conference on contemporary computing and informatics (IC3I), Mysuru, India. IEEE, pp 1135–1139
4. Le TH, Caracoglia L (2015) Rectangular prism pressure coherence by modified Morlet continuous wavelet transform. Wind Struct 20(5):661–682
5. Saatlo AN, Ozoguz S (2015) CMOS implementation of scalable Morlet wavelet for application in signal processing. In: 38th international conference on telecommunications and signal processing (TSP), Prague, Czech Republic. IEEE, pp 4–9
6. Mousavi SA, Hanifeloo Z, Sumari P, Arshad MRM (2016) Enhancing the diagnosis of corn pests using Gabor wavelet features and SVM classification. J Sci Ind Res 75(6):349–354
7. Lu HM (2016) Facial emotion recognition based on biorthogonal wavelet entropy, fuzzy support vector machine, and stratified cross validation. IEEE Access 4:8375–8385. https://doi.org/10.1109/ACCESS.2016.2628407
8. Zhan TM, Chen Y (2016) Multiple sclerosis detection based on biorthogonal wavelet transform, RBF kernel principal component analysis, and logistic regression. IEEE Access 4:7567–7576. https://doi.org/10.1109/ACCESS.2016.2620996
9. Postnikov EB, Singh VK (2015) Continuous wavelet transform with the Shannon wavelet from the point of view of hyperbolic partial differential equations. Anal Math 41(3):199–206. https://doi.org/10.1007/s10476-015-0206-2
10. Abidin ZZ, Manaf M, Shibhgatullah AS (2013) Experimental approach on thresholding using reverse biorthogonal wavelet decomposition for eye image. In: International conference on signal and image processing applications, Melaka, Malaysia. IEEE, pp 349–353
11. Boufares O, Aloui N, Cherif A (2016) Adaptive threshold for background subtraction in moving object detection using stationary wavelet transforms 2D. Int J Adv Comput Sci Appl 7(8):29–36
12. Juneau PM, Garnier A, Duchesne C (2015) The undecimated wavelet transform-multivariate image analysis (UWT-MIA) for simultaneous extraction of spectral and spatial information. Chemometr Intell Lab Syst 142:304–318. https://doi.org/10.1016/j.chemolab.2014.09.007
13. Kumar A, Sunkaria RK (2016) Two-channel perfect reconstruction (PR) quadrature mirror filter (QMF) bank design using logarithmic window function and spline function. SIViP 10 (8):1473–1480. https://doi.org/10.1007/s11760-016-0958-6
14. Li Y (2016) Detection of dendritic spines using wavelet packet entropy and fuzzy support vector machine. CNS Neurol Disord: Drug Targets 15:116–121. https://doi.org/10.2174/1871527315666161111123638
15. Yang J (2015) Preclinical diagnosis of magnetic resonance (MR) brain images via discrete wavelet packet transform with Tsallis entropy and generalized eigenvalue proximal support vector machine (GEPSVM). Entropy 17(4):1795–1813. https://doi.org/10.3390/e17041795
16. Yang M (2016) Dual-tree complex wavelet transform and twin support vector machine for pathological brain detection. Appl Sci 6(6), Article ID: 169
17. Lama RK, Choi MR, Kwon GR (2016) Image interpolation for high-resolution display based on the complex dual-tree wavelet transform and hidden Markov model. Multimedia Tools Appl 75(23):16487–16498. https://doi.org/10.1007/s11042-016-3245-1
18. Fahmy MF, Fahmy OM (2016) An enhanced denoising technique using dual tree complex wavelet transform. In: El Khamy S, El Badawy H, El Diasty S (eds), 33rd national radio science conference NRSC, Aswan, Egypt. IEEE, pp 205–211
19. Canbay F, Levent VE, Serbes G, Fatih Ugurdag H, Goren S, Aydin N (2016) A multi-channel real time implementation of dual tree complex wavelet transform in field programmable gate arrays. In: Kyriacou E, Christofides S, Pattichis C (eds) XIV mediterranean conference on medical and biological engineering and computing 2016. IFMBE proceedings, vol 57. Springer, Cham, pp 114–118. https://doi.org/10.1007/978-3-319-32703-7_24

Chapter 7
Dimensionality Reduction of Brain Image Features

If the feature number is too large, it causes the curse of the dimensionality problem. In the pathological brain detection (PBD) system, each feature may have many possible values. Therefore, to ensure several samples exist with each combination of different feature values, an enormous amount of training data is required. Otherwise, if the training samples number is fixed, the classification performance deteriorates as the feature number increases. In a word, dimensionality reduction (DR) is necessary to reduce the feature number. DR is divided into two categories: feature selection and feature extraction. For the former, filter, wrapper, and embedded methods are introduced. In addition, three important filter methods are discussed: student's t-test, Welch's t-test, and Bhattacharyya distance. For the latter, principal component analysis and its variants (kernel principal component analysis and probabilistic principal component analysis) are provided. Finally, an introduction and a through comparison of the autoencoder, denoising autoencoder, and sparse autoencoder are provided.

7.1 Feature Selection

Feature selection is aimed at finding a subset of the original features. Three types of feature selection methods exist, based on how the selection algorithm and model building are combined. Figure 7.1 shows these three types. Table 7.1 lists their advantages and disadvantages. They are briefly described here:

- Filter methods analyze the intrinsic properties of the features, while neglecting the classifier [1]. It first evaluates each individual feature, ignoring their interactions. Then, it ranks the individual features and chooses a subset.
- Wrapper methods evaluate subsets of features and detect their potential interactions [2]. While the number of observations is insufficient, the risk of overfitting increases.

© Springer Nature Singapore Pte Ltd. 2018
S.-H. Wang et al., *Pathological Brain Detection*, Brain Informatics and Health,
https://doi.org/10.1007/978-981-10-4026-9_7

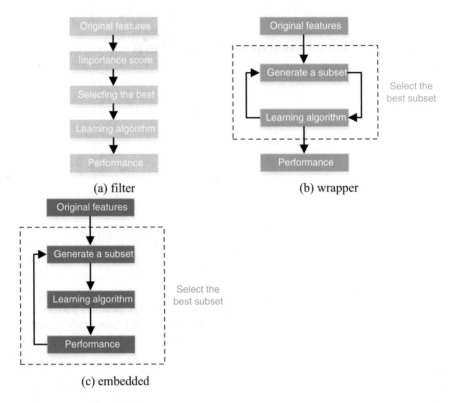

(a) filter

(b) wrapper

(c) embedded

Fig. 7.1 Three types of feature selection

Table 7.1 Comparison of feature selection methods

Type	Advantages	Disadvantages
Filter	Fast execution and robust to overfitting	May select redundant variables
Wrapper	High accuracy	Slow execution and susceptible to overfitting
Embedded	Combination of filters and wrappers	Selection procedure needs to be identified in advance

- Embedded methods combined the advantages of both filters and wrappers [3]. The learning algorithms make full use of the selection algorithm, hence, its disadvantage is determining the selection criterion and search algorithm beforehand.

7.2 Several Filter Methods

Filter type methods select variables regardless of the model. They are based only on general features like the correlation with the variable chosen to predict.

7.2.1 Student's t-Test

Student's t-test (STT) [4] is regarded as one of the filters, since it measures the degree of difference of features over two classes. STT is the most popular method that assumes "equal means" and "equal variances" of the two data sets. Due to the unequal sample sizes, the STT is computed by:

$$s(p,q) = \frac{\mu_p - \mu_q}{\sqrt{\frac{(n_p-1)\sigma_p^2 + (n_q-1)\sigma_q^2}{n_p + n_q - 2}} \sqrt{\frac{1}{n_p} + \frac{1}{n_q}}} \tag{7.1}$$

where s is the STT score and n the sample size.

The STT can be performed using the "ttest" command in Matlab software. The command details are listed in Table 7.2.

7.2.2 Welch's t-Test

"Equal variances" does not make sense and can be discarded; the "equal means" is necessary. We use Welch's t-test (WTT), an adaption of the STT [5]. WTT only checks whether the two populations have equal means, it is computed by:

Table 7.2 The "ttest" command

[h,p,ci,stats] = ttest(x, y)
Input: x: sample data   y: sample data   (x, y) must be the same size.
Output: h: Hypothesis test result   p: p-value   ci: confidence interval   stats: test statistics[a]

[a]Including the degree of freedom of the test, and the estimated population standard deviation

$$w(p,q) = \frac{\mu_p - \mu_q}{\sqrt{\frac{\sigma_p^2}{n_p} + \frac{\sigma_q^2}{n_q}}} \tag{7.2}$$

where μ denotes the sample mean; σ^2 the variance; n the sample size; and w the WTT score. The null hypothesis in this work is that a specific feature of the two classes have the same means (equal variances are not considered). The alternative hypothesis is that they have unequal means.

7.2.3 Bhattacharyya Distance

The Bhattacharyya distance (BD) measures the relative closeness of two discrete (or continuous) probability distributions [6]. Suppose the data of two classes fall under the normal distribution, the BD is formed as:

$$b(p,q) = \frac{1}{4} \times \ln\left(\left(\frac{\sigma_p^2}{\sigma_q^2} + \frac{\sigma_q^2}{\sigma_p^2} + 2\right)/4\right) + \frac{1}{4} \times \left(\frac{(\mu_p - \mu_q)^2}{\sigma_p^2 + \sigma_q^2}\right) \tag{7.3}$$

where μ denotes the sample mean; σ^2 the variance; and p and q represent two classes. Compared to the Mahalanobis distance (MD) [7], the BD is more reliable since the MD is a particular case of the BD when the standard deviations of the two classes are equal.

7.3 Feature Extraction

Feature extraction transforms original features into a reduced set of features. The transformation can be either linear or nonlinear. The main linear technique is principal component analysis (PCA) [8], which maps original features to low-dimensional space in the way that the variance of a transformed feature is maximized. Kernel PCA [9] is an extension of PCA and is capable of constructing nonlinear mappings.

Some nonlinear methods can be viewed as defining a graph-based kernel for PCA. These methods include isomap [10], Laplacian eigenmap, locally linear embedding (LLE) [11], etc. These techniques generate a low-dimensional transformed feature via a cost function, and retain the local properties of the original feature.

Semidefinite embedding (SDE) learns the kernel using semidefinite programing instead of using fixed kernels. It first creates a neighborhood graph, where each input feature is connected with its k-nearest input features and all k-nearest neighbors are fully connected with each other. Next, the semidefinite programing aims to find an inner product matrix that maximizes the pairwise distances between any two inputs that are not connected.

An autoencoder is a feed-forward, non-recurrent neural network used to learn a representation for a set of features [12]. The output layer of an autoencoder has the same number of nodes as in the input layer [13]. Instead of being trained to target values in the traditional neural network, an autoencoder is trained to reconstruct their own input features. Therefore, autoencoders can be used for DR. Section 7.5 outlines how to instruct an autoencoder.

7.4 Principal Component Analysis

As an effective DR tool, PCA can reduce the size of wavelet coefficients from magnetic resonance (MR) brain images [14].

7.4.1 Mathematical Form

Assume there is a data set C with size N and dimension d, first we calculate the sample mean m_j of the jth feature as:

$$m_j = \frac{1}{N} \times \sum_{i=1}^{N} C(i,j) \tag{7.4}$$

Next, we calculate the zero-mean data set B as:

$$B = C - em^T \tag{7.5}$$

Here e represents an $N \times 1$ vector of all ones.

Third, the $d \times d$ covariance matrix Z is generated:

$$Z = \frac{B^*B}{N-1} \tag{7.6}$$

Fourth, the covariance matrix Z has an eigen decomposition expression as:

$$Z = XYX^{-1} \tag{7.7}$$

Here X represents the eigenvector matrix and Y represents the eigenvalue matrix, which is also a diagonal matrix:

$$Y = \begin{bmatrix} Y(1,1) & & & \\ & Y(2,2) & & \\ & & \ddots & \\ & & & Y(d,d) \end{bmatrix} \tag{7.8}$$

Fifth, we rearrange X and Y, so that the eigenvalue is decreasing:

$$Y(1,1) \geq Y(2,2) \geq \cdots \geq Y(d,d) \tag{7.9}$$

Sixth, we calculate cumulative variance for each eigenvector by:

$$G(k) = \sum_{i=1}^{k} Y(i,i) \tag{7.10}$$

Thus, we can form a vector as:

$$G = \begin{bmatrix} G(1) & G(2) & \cdots & G(d) \end{bmatrix} \tag{7.11}$$

Seventh, assume the threshold is T, and thus we select L^* which satisfies:

$$L^* = \arg\min\left\{ L \left| \frac{G(L)}{G(d)} \geq T \right. \right\} \tag{7.12}$$

Finally, the most important principal components (PCs) of L^* are output [15]. Figure 7.2 shows an example, where two PCs are generated from hundreds of points.

Table 7.3 details Matlab's "pca" command, which allows calculation of PC coefficients, scores, variances, and other statistics.

7.4.2 Kernel Principal Component Analysis

One shortcoming of PCA is that it cannot extract nonlinear structure information [16]. To solve this problem, scholars have proposed a powerful variant of PCA—kernel PCA (KPCA) [17]. KPCA does the same as PCA except it transforms the data set C into a higher dimensional space [18].

Two different KPCAs have been studied. One is the polynomial KPCA (PKPCA) defined as:

$$k(x, y | \text{PKPCA}) = (a(x \times y) + b)^c \tag{7.13}$$

where a, b, and c are kernel parameters.

The other is RBF KPCA (RKPCA) [19] defined as:

Fig. 7.2 Two PCs generated by PCA

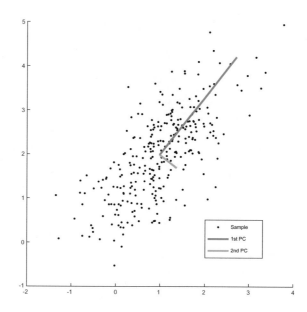

Table 7.3 The "pca" command

[coeff, score, latent, tsquared, exp, mu] = pca(X)
Input x: input matrix
Output coeff: PC coefficients score: PC scores latent: PC variances tsquared: Hotelling's T-squared statistic exp: Percentage of total variance explained mu: estimated means

$$k(x, y|\text{RKPCA}) = \exp\left(-\frac{\|x - y\|^2}{d^2}\right) \qquad (7.14)$$

where d represents the scaling factor.

The optimal estimation of hyperparameters a, b, c, and d can be obtained using a grid search (GS) algorithm [20]. GS is also named parameter sweep. It is an exhaustive searching method within a manually specified subset of hyperparameter space. Random search may be an alternative way to accelerate finding the optimal values of these hyperparameters.

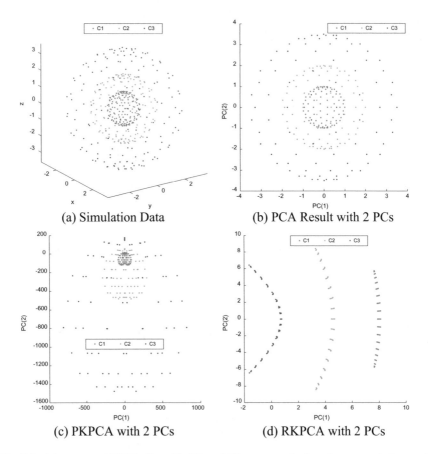

(a) Simulation Data   (b) PCA Result with 2 PCs

(c) PKPCA with 2 PCs   (d) RKPCA with 2 PCs

Fig. 7.3 Advantages of KPCA. *Note* C1, C2, and C3 represent the first class, second class, and third class, respectively

7.4.3   Advantages of Kernel Principal Component Analysis

We generate sample points of three classes in Fig. 7.3a. All points lie in spheres with different radii. Figure 7.3b shows PCA results and Fig. 7.3c shows PKPCA results. The results suggest that the two PCs selected by either PCA or PKPCA cannot segment different classes. Figure 7.3d shows RKPCA results, which indicate that even one PC selected by RKPCA can segment the three classes.

7.4.4   Probabilistic Principal Component Analysis

Probabilistic principal component analysis (PPCA) estimates the principal axes and principal components [21] for any data vector which has missing values. It is based on an isotropic error model as:

Table 7.4 The "ppca" command

[coeff, score, pcvar, mu, v, S] = ppca(Y, K)
Input: Y: input data K: number of PCs
Output: coeff: PC coefficients score: PC scores pcvar: PC variances mu: estimated mean v: isotropic residue variance S: final results at convergence

$$y = Wx + \mu + \varepsilon \tag{7.15}$$

where x is the unobserved (latent) vector; y is the observed vector; W relates x and y; μ permits the model to have a nonzero mean; and ε is the isotropic error term with:

$$\varepsilon \sim N(0, v * I(k)) \tag{7.16}$$

where v is the residual variance and k should be smaller than the rank for $v > 0$. For PPCA, the model of the observed vector is:

$$y \sim N(\mu, W * W^T + v * I(k)) \tag{7.17}$$

The solution of W and v are commonly completed using an expectation–maximization (EM) algorithm [22]. The advantages of PPCA over standard PCA is two-fold [23]:

1. PCA is the limiting case of PPCA, where v is equal to zero.
2. PPCA can handle missing values through the data set.

PPCA can be carried out in Matlab using the "ppca" command. The meanings of input and out parameters are listed in Table 7.4.

7.5   Autoencoder

An autoencoder (AE), also called an auto-associator, is an artificial neural network that can learn efficient coding for unlabeled data [24]. An AE can be used for dimensionality reduction [25]. The structure of an AE is a feed-forward, non-recurrent network with input layer, several hidden layers (typically one), and one output layer [26]. The output layer Y has the same number of nodes as the input layer X.

Fig. 7.4 Structure of an AE. *Note X*, input vector; *Y*, output vector; *E* weight matrix of encoder part; *D*, the weight matrix of decoder part; *A*, output of hidden neuron

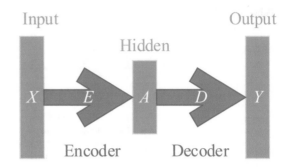

Figure 7.4 shows the structure of an AE with one hidden layer *A*. The AE is trained so that the output *Y* is approximate to the input *X*. The AE can be divided into encoder *E* and decoder *D*, where:

$$E : X \rightarrow A \qquad (7.18)$$

$$D : A \rightarrow Y \qquad (7.19)$$

The training is to simplify the following loss function:

$$\underset{D,E}{\arg\min} \|X - Y\|^2 \qquad (7.20)$$

where *Y* is defined as:

$$Y = D(E(X)) \qquad (7.21)$$

Table 7.5 presents the input and output arguments of Matlab's "trainAutoencoder" command. The purpose of this command is to train an AE.

7.5.1 Denoising Autoencoder

A denoising autoencoder (DAE) takes partially corrupted input, while training to recover the original clean input [27]. A DAE is one of the techniques of good representation, which can be obtained robustly from corrupted input.

Table 7.5 The "trainAutoencoder" command

autoenc = trainAutoencoder(X, hs)
Input X: training data hs: Size of hidden representation of the autoencoder
Output autoenc: trained autoencoder

To train a DAE, we need to perform preliminary stochastic mapping:

$$X \to \tilde{X} \tag{7.22}$$

Therefore, the corrupted input $\tilde{X}$ is used to input into a normal AE. The training procedure is performed using the scaled conjugate gradient descent (SCGD) method.

7.5.2 Sparse Autoencoder

The sparse autoencoder (SAE) imposes sparsity on the hidden units during training. This allows sparse representation of the inputs [28]. The SAE is commonly used for the pretraining of a classification task [29]. Sparsity is often achieved by additional terms in the loss function, or by manually zeroing all but the strongest hidden unit activations [30].

To minimize the error between the input vector X and output Y, we can yield the objective function as:

$$J(E, D, B_1, B_2) = \frac{1}{2} \|Y - X\|^2 \tag{7.23}$$

We can deduce that Y can be expressed as:

$$Y = h(X|E, D, B_1, B_2) \tag{7.24}$$

Hence, Eq. (7.23) can be revised as:

$$J(E, D, B_1, B_2) = \frac{1}{2} \|h(X|E, D, B_1, B_2) - X\|^2 \tag{7.25}$$

To avoid over-complete mapping or learn trivial mapping, we add one regularization term on the weight and one regularization term of a sparse constraint:

$$J(E, D, B_1, B_2) = \frac{1}{2} \|h(X|E, D, B_1, B_2) - X\|^2 \\ + \alpha \sum_j K(\rho, \rho_j) + \beta \| E \quad D \|_2^2 \tag{7.26}$$

where α is the weight of the sparse penalty and β the regularization factor controlling the degree of weight decay. $K(\ )$ is the Kullback–Leibler divergence [31, 32] defined as:

$$K(a,b) = a \times \log\frac{a}{b} + (1-a) \times \log\frac{1-a}{1-b} \qquad (7.27)$$

The symbol ρ represents the desired probability of being activated and ρ_j the average activation probability of the jth hidden neuron.

7.6 Conclusion

This chapter describes several typical DR techniques. These methods are crucial, due to the "curse of dimensionality" problem. For very high–dimensional data sets, readers may refer to some other specific toolboxes.

References

1. Ambusaidi MA, He XJ, Nanda P, Tan ZY (2016) Building an intrusion detection system using a filter-based feature selection algorithm. IEEE Trans Comput 65(10):2986–2998. https://doi.org/10.1109/tc.2016.2519914
2. Das S, Singh PK, Bhowmik S, Sarkar R, Nasipuri M (2016) A harmony search based wrapper feature selection method for Holistic Bangla word recognition. In: Venugopal KR, Buyya R, Patnaik LM, Shenoy PD, Iyengar SS, Raja KB (eds) Twelfth international conference on communication networks (ICCN), Bangalore, India. Procedia computer science. Elsevier Science Bv, pp 395–403. https://doi.org/10.1016/j.procs.2016.06.087
3. Silvestre C, Cardoso M, Figueiredo M (2015) Feature selection for clustering categorical data with an embedded modelling approach. Expert Syst 32(3):444–453. https://doi.org/10.1111/exsy.12082
4. Stetten G, Horvath S, Galeotti J, Shukla G, Wang B, Chapman B. (2010) Image segmentation using the student's t-test and the divergence of direction on spherical regions. In: Dawant BM, Haynor DR (eds) Medical imaging 2010: image processing, vol 7623. Proceedings of SPIE. SPIE, Bellingham, pp 342–347. https://doi.org/10.1117/12.844014
5. Ahad NA, Yahaya SSS (2014) Sensitivity analysis of Welch's t-Test. In: Ismail MT, Ahmad S, Rahman RA (eds) Proceedings of the 21st national symposium on mathematical sciences, Malaysia. AIP Conference Proceedings. American Institute of Physics, pp 888–893. https://doi.org/10.1063/1.4887707
6. So RWK, Chung ACS (2017) A novel learning-based dissimilarity metric for rigid and non-rigid medical image registration by using Bhattacharyya distances. Pattern Recogn 62:161–174. https://doi.org/10.1016/j.patcog.2016.09.004
7. Gonzalez-Arteaga T, Alcantud JCR, Calle RD (2016) A new consensus ranking approach for correlated ordinal information based on Mahalanobis distance. Inf Sci 372:546–564. https://doi.org/10.1016/j.ins.2016.08.071
8. Mudali D, Teune LK, Renken RJ, Leenders KL, Roerdink J (2015) Classification of Parkinsonian syndromes from FDG-PET brain data using decision trees with SSM/PCA features. Comput Math Methods Med, Article ID: 136921. https://doi.org/10.1155/2015/136921
9. Washizawa Y (2016) Learning subspace classification using subset approximated kernel principal component analysis. IEICE Trans Inf Syst E99D(5):1353–1363. https://doi.org/10.1587/transinf.2015EDP7334

10. Krivov E, Belyaev M (2016) Dimensionality reduction with isomap algorithm for EEG covariance matrices. In: 4th international winter conference on brain-computer interface (BCI), South Korea. IEEE, p 4

11. Nguyen V, Hung CC, Ma X (2015) Super resolution face image based on locally linear embedding and local correlation. Appl Comput Rev 15(1):17–25. https://doi.org/10.1145/2663761.2663767

12. Lore KG, Akintayo A, Sarkar S (2017) LLNet: a deep autoencoder approach to natural low-light image enhancement. Pattern Recogn 61:650–662. https://doi.org/10.1016/j.patcog.2016.06.008

13. Potapov A, Potapova V, Peterson M (2016) A feasibility study of an autoencoder meta-model for improving generalization capabilities on training sets of small sizes. Pattern Recogn Lett 80:24–29. https://doi.org/10.1016/j.patrec.2016.05.018

14. Chen Y, Chen X-Q (2016) Sensorineural hearing loss detection via discrete wavelet transform and principal component analysis combined with generalized eigenvalue proximal support vector machine and Tikhonov regularization. Multimedia Tools Appl. https://doi.org/10.1007/s11042-016-4087-6

15. Sharma S, Vinuchakravarthy S, Subramanian SJ (2017) Estimation of surface curvature from full-field shape data using principal component analysis. Meas Sci Technol 28(1), Article ID: 015003. https://doi.org/10.1088/0957-0233/28/1/015003

16. Zhan TM, Chen Y (2016) Multiple sclerosis detection based on biorthogonal wavelet transform, RBF kernel principal component analysis, and logistic regression. IEEE Access 4:7567–7576. https://doi.org/10.1109/ACCESS.2016.2620996

17. Sheng JL, Dong SJ, Liu Z, Gao HW (2016) Fault feature extraction method based on local mean decomposition Shannon entropy and improved kernel principal component analysis model. Adv Mech Eng 8(8), Article ID: 1687814016661087. https://doi.org/10.1177/1687814016661087

18. Duan XF, Qi PY, Tian Z (2016) Registration for variform object of remote-sensing image using improved robust weighted kernel principal component analysis. J Indian Soc Remote Sens 44(5):675–686. https://doi.org/10.1007/s12524-015-0545-2

19. Joseph AA, Tokumoto T, Ozawa S (2016) Online feature extraction based on accelerated kernel principal component analysis for data stream. Evolving Syst 7(1):15–27. https://doi.org/10.1007/s12530-015-9131-7

20. Hafezi S, Moore AH, Naylor PA (2016) Multiple source localization in the spherical harmonic domain using augmented intensity vectors based on grid search. In: 24th european signal processing conference (EUSIPCO), Budapest, Hungary. IEEE, pp 602–606. https://doi.org/10.1109/eusipco.2016.7760319

21. Nyamundanda G, Brennan L, Gormley IC (2010) Probabilistic principal component analysis for metabolomic data. BMC Bioinform 11(1):571–561. https://doi.org/10.1186/1471-2105-11-571

22. Sadeghian A, Huang B (2016) Robust probabilistic principal component analysis for process modeling subject to scaled mixture Gaussian noise. Comput Chem Eng 90:62–78. https://doi.org/10.1016/j.compchemeng.2016.03.031

23. Mredhula L, Dorairangaswamy MA (2016) An effective filtering technique for image denoising using probabilistic principal component analysis (PPCA). J Med Imaging Health Inform 6(1):194–203. https://doi.org/10.1166/jmihi.2016.1602

24. Gupta P, Banchs RE, Rosso P (2016) Squeezing bottlenecks: exploring the limits of autoencoder semantic representation capabilities. Neurocomputing 175:1001–1008. https://doi.org/10.1016/j.neucom.2015.06.091

25. Saha M, Mitra P, Nanjundiah RS (2016) Autoencoder-based identification of predictors of Indian monsoon. Meteorol Atmos Phys 128(5):613–628. https://doi.org/10.1007/s00703-016-0431-7

26. Ueda Y, Wang LB, Kai A, Xiao X, Chng ES, Li HZ (2016) Single-channel dereverberation for distant-talking speech recognition by combining denoising autoencoder and temporal

structure normalization. J Signal Process Syst Signal Image Video Technol 82(2):151–161. https://doi.org/10.1007/s11265-015-1007-3

27. Moubayed N, Breckon T, Matthews P, McGough AS (2016) SMS spam filtering using probabilistic topic modelling and stacked denoising autoencoder. In: Villa AEP, Masulli P, Rivero AJP (eds) 25th international conference on artificial neural networks (ICANN), Barcelona, Spain. Lecture Notes in Computer Science. Springer International Publishing AG, pp 423–430. https://doi.org/10.1007/978-3-319-44781-0_50

28. Kim HC, Lee JH (2016) Evaluation of weight sparsity control during autoencoder training of resting-state fMRI using non-zero ratio and Hoyer's sparseness. In: 6th international workshop on pattern recognition in neuroimaging, Trento, Italy. International workshop on pattern recognition in neuroimaging. IEEE, pp 121–124

29. Furuya T, Ohbuchi R (2016) Accurate aggregation of local features by using K-sparse autoencoder for 3D model retrieval. In: ACM international conference on multimedia retrieval, New York City, NY. ACM, pp 293–297. https://doi.org/10.1145/2911996.2912054

30. Utkin LV, Popov SG, Zhuk YA (2016) Robust transfer learning in multi-robot systems by using sparse autoencoder. In: Xix international conference on soft computing and measurements (SCM 2016), St Petersburg, Russia. IEEE, pp 224–227

31. Raitoharju M, Garcia-Fernandez AF, Piche R (2017) Kullback-Leibler divergence approach to partitioned update Kalman filter. Signal Process 130:289–298. https://doi.org/10.1016/j.sigpro.2016.07.007

32. Nielsen F, Sun K (2016) Guaranteed Bounds on the Kullback-Leibler divergence of univariate mixtures. IEEE Signal Process Lett 23(11):1543–1546. https://doi.org/10.1109/lsp.2016.2606661

Chapter 8
Classification Methods for Pathological Brain Detection

In PBD systems, classification entails identifying which disease category a new magnetic resonance (MR) image belongs to. This chapter first describes four pre-design tasks: the trade-off between bias and variance, data volume and classifier complexity, noise at the target, and the class imbalance problem. Further to this, three canonical classifiers: the naive Bayesian classifier, the decision tree (trained by ID3 and C4.5), and k-nearest neighbors, are discussed. Two variants of this last classifier are analyzed: one-nearest neighbor and weighted nearest neighbor. The support vector machine is extremely important in both PBD and other applications. Its mathematical fundamentals are analyzed. The generalized eigenvalue proximal support vector machine, twin support vector machine, and fuzzy support vector machine are expatiated. The multiclass technique to generalize the support vector machine for multiclass problems is provided. The feed-forward neural network is introduced with an explanation given about constructing the encoding strategy and criterion. Three activation functions are compared. Besides this, three variants of feed-forward neural networks are presented, that is, the extreme learning machine, the radial basis function network, and the probabilistic neural network. Finally, the linear regression classifier (LRC) is introduced and analyzed.

8.1 Pre-design Tasks

8.1.1 Trade-off Between Bias and Variance

Classification performance is related to both the bias and variance of the learning algorithm over several given data sets. A learning algorithm with low bias should be versatile to other data sets. Hence, a good learning algorithm should balance bias and variance automatically.

© Springer Nature Singapore Pte Ltd. 2018
S.-H. Wang et al., *Pathological Brain Detection*, Brain Informatics and Health,
https://doi.org/10.1007/978-981-10-4026-9_8

8.1.2   Data Volume and Classifier Complexity

If the classifier is complicated, then it will learn from an exceptionally large data set with low bias and high variance. In contrast, a simple classifier will learn from a small volume of training data with high bias and low variance. Therefore, a learning algorithm should adjust itself, taking into consideration both the data volume and its structural complexity.

8.1.3   Noise at the Target

Targets may be incorrect, since neuroradiologists may mislabel brain images. This suggests that a learning algorithm does not need to match the training data exactly. Noise at the target can be modeled as deterministic noise and can be alleviated by "overfitting prevention" techniques.

In this book, noise at the target means that an incorrect diagnosis might be made when using images, as shown in Fig. 8.1. Hence, it is necessary to detect and remove mislabeled brain images.

8.1.4   Class-Imbalance Problem

It is easy to obtain brain images from healthy controls, but it is quite difficult to acquire MR images from patients, particularly uncooperative patients. The medical

Fig. 8.1 The human expert may make errors

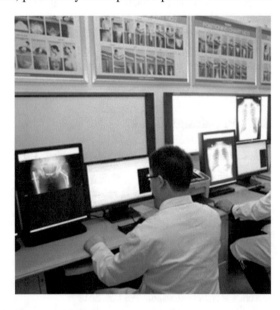

diagnosis data set rarely contains positive observations and often numerous negative ones. This leads to low sensitivity and high specificity. Several techniques can
be used to alleviate the class imbalance problem, such as resampling [1],
cost-sensitive boosting, cost-sensitive learning, ensemble, etc.

8.2   Naive Bayesian Classifier

The naive Bayes classifier (NBC) is widely recognized as a simple probabilistic
classifier based on the application of the Bayesian theorem with strong (naive)
independence assumptions.

An NBC considers each of the input features to contribute independently to the
probability, regardless of the presence or absence of other features. In spite of their
naive design and apparently oversimplified assumptions, they works quite well in
various complicated real-world situations [2].

For some types of probability models, NBCs can be trained very efficiently in a
supervised learning setting. In many practical applications, parameter estimation for
NBC uses the method of maximum likelihood.

The probability model for an NBC is a conditional model over a dependent class
variable C with a small number of outcomes or classes, conditional on several
feature variables X_1 through X_n:

$$p(C|X_1, X_2, \ldots, X_n) \tag{8.1}$$

However, if a feature can take on a large number of values or if the number of
features n is too large, then basing such a model on probability tables is infeasible.
We therefore reformulate the model to make it more tractable:

$$p(C|X_1, X_2, \ldots, X_n) = \frac{p(C)p(X_1, X_2, \ldots, X_n|C)}{p(X_1, X_2, \ldots, X_n)} \tag{8.2}$$

In Bayesian analysis, the final classification is produced by combining both
sources of information, prior and likelihood [3], to form a posterior probability
using the so-called Bayes' rule.

In practice, there is interest only in the numerator of that fraction, because the
denominator does not depend on C and the values of the features X_i are given, so
that the denominator is effectively constant. Therefore, we just need to maximize
the value of:

$$p(C)p(X_1, X_2, \ldots, X_n|C) \tag{8.3}$$

Now the "naïve" conditional independence assumptions come into play: assume
that each feature X_i is conditionally independent of every other feature X_j for $j \neq i$,
given the category C:

Table 8.1 The "fitcnb" command	**Mdl = fitcnb(X, Y)**
	Input X: predictor data Y: class labels
	Output Mdl: trained naive Bayes classification model

$$p(X_1, X_2, \ldots, X_n | C) = \prod_{i=1}^{n} p(X_i | C) \qquad (8.4)$$

where the probability $p(X_1|C)$, ..., $p(X_n|C)$ can be estimated using the training sample.

Through these calculations, we can obtain the posterior probabilities of a sample belonging to each class. Finally, we select the class with the largest posterior probability as a class label, based on Bayesian maximum a posteriori criteria.

Table 8.1 details Matlab's "fitcnb" command which can implement the training of an NBC model.

8.3 Decision Tree

A decision tree (DT) [4] is a tree-like structure (Fig. 8.2). Each node represents a test over an attribute, each branch denotes its outcome, and each leaf node denotes a class label. The path from root node to leaf node can be seen as a classification rule. The goal of the learning method for a DT is to create a DT model that predicts the value of a target class label, on the basis of input attributes.

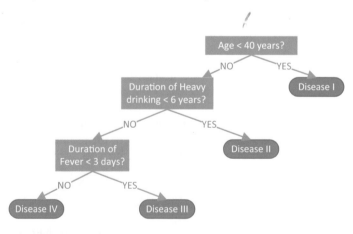

Fig. 8.2 An example of a decision tree

Table 8.2 The "fitctree" command

tree = fitctree(X,Y)
Input X: predictor data Y: class labels
Output tree: trained tree

The training of a DT can be accomplished using Matlab's "fitctree" command, detailed in Table 8.2.

8.3.1 ID3 Algorithm

The ID3 algorithm begins with the original set S as the root node. It iterates through all unused attributes in the set S, and calculates the entropy or information gain (IG) of that attribute. It then selects the attribute with the smallest entropy or IG. The set S is split by the selected attribute to produce subsets of the data. ID3 continues to recurse on each subset, only considering unselected attributes.

8.3.2 C4.5 Algorithm

C4.5 is an extension of the ID3 algorithm [5]. C4.5 chooses, at each node, the attribute that most effectively splits the samples into subsets that were enriched in one class or the other. The IG can be chosen as the splitting criterion. The attribute with the largest normalized IG is tested to prove the algorithm is useful. Then, the C4.5 is then repeated on smaller sub-lists.

8.3.3 Classification and Regression Tree

The classification and regression tree (CART) [6] is a non-parametric learning technique for a decision tree. It can produce both a classification tree and a regression tree, depending on whether the response variable is categoric or numeric [7].

Initially, CART selects rules to obtain the best split, so as to differentiate samples based on the dependent variables. This process is applied to each child node recursively, until CART detects no further gain or until some predefined termination criterion is met.

8.3.4 Ensemble Methods

Ensemble methods are usually employed to construct a collection of decision trees, e.g., random forest (RF), gradient tree boosting (GTB), and bagging tree. Table 8.3 shows their implementation methods.

8.4 *k*-Nearest Neighbors

For the k-nearest neighbors (kNN) algorithm, the input contains k closest training data, and the output is a class membership [8], by which a new instance is assigned to the class that is most common to its k neighbors [9].

Figure 8.3 shows an example of the kNN algorithm, where the new instance (a blue circle) should be classified as being in the class of red squares, because there are three red squares and two black diamonds within the dashed circle.

kNN is a type of lazy learning, i.e., all computation is deferred until the new-instance classification stage [10]. In this binary classification problem, it is beneficial to set k to an odd number, so as to avoid tied votes. The bootstrap method can be used to set the optimal value of k. Euclidean distance can then be employed to measure the distance. Table 8.4 details Matlab's "fitcknn" command, which can be used to fit the kNN classifier.

Table 8.3 Three typical ensemble methods for constructing decision trees

Name	Method
Random forest	It uses a number of decision trees in order to improve the classification rate
Gradient tree boosting	It uses gradient boosting as a fix-sized base learner. It can be used for both regression-type and classification-type problems
Bagging tree	It is an early ensemble method, building multiple trees by repeatedly resampling training data with replacement, and majority voting for a consensus

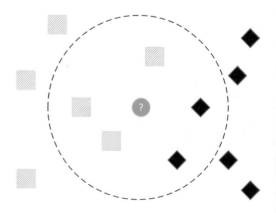

Fig. 8.3 An example showing the principle behind the kNN algorithm

Table 8.4 The "fitcknn" command	**Mdl = fitcknn(X,Y)**
	Input X: predictor data Y: class labels
	Output Mdl: trained kNN model

8.4.1   One-Nearest Neighbor

The most intuitive kNN is the one-nearest neighbor (ONN) [11] classifier, which assigns a new sample to the class of its closest neighboring sample. As the size of training data set increases to infinity, the ONN converges to an error rate of no worse than twice the Bayes error rate (BER).

Note that the BER denotes the lowest possible error rate for any classifier of a random outcome. It can be viewed as the irreducible error.

8.4.2   Weighted Nearest Neighbor

The kNN can be regarded as assigning k nearest neighbors a weight of $1/k$ and all other neighbors a weight of 0. This idea yields the weighted nearest neighbor (WNN) classifier, which assigns the ith nearest neighbor a weight w_i with:

$$\sum_{i=1}^{k} w_i = 1 \tag{8.5}$$

Compared to the standard kNN, the introduction of weights improves the classification performance. The reason for this is that the training samples that are nearer to the objects are more similar to each other, so they are more likely to be classified in the same class. Therefore, the classification performance of the WNN is usually better than the standard kNN.

8.5   Support Vector Machine

Given a set of two-category training examples, a support vector machine (SVM) training algorithm builds a model that assigns new examples to one category or the other, making it a non-probabilistic binary linear classifier.

Suppose there is a p-dimensional N-point training data set. The data set can be formulated as:

$$\{(x_i, y_i) | x_i \in R^p, y_i \in \{-1, +1\}\}, i = 1, 2, 3, \dots, N \qquad (8.6)$$

here x denotes a p-dimensional training point and y_i is either -1 or $+1$th, denoting at the sample can be in class 1 or class 2. The aim is to generate a $(p-1)$-dimensional hyperplane as:

$$\mathbf{w}x - \mathbf{b} = 0 \qquad (8.7)$$

Here $\mathbf{w}$ and $\mathbf{b}$ denote the weights and biases. Their values are optimized with the criterion to maximize the distance between the two hyperplanes that are parallel, while still separating the data:

$$\min_{b,\mathbf{w}} \|\mathbf{w}\|^2 / 2$$
$$\text{s.t.} y_i(\mathbf{w}x_i - \mathbf{b}) \geq 1, \, i = 1, 2, 3, \dots, N \qquad (8.8)$$

Figure 8.4 shows an SVM over a 2D data set. Positive slack vectors $\xi = (\xi_1, \dots, \xi_n, \dots, \xi_N)$ are added to measure the misclassification degree of sample p_n. Hence, the mathematical formula of the optimal SVM can be deduced by solving:

$$\min_{\mathbf{w}, \xi, \mathbf{b}} \frac{1}{2} \|\mathbf{w}\|^2 + Le^T \xi$$
$$\text{s.t.} \begin{cases} y_n(\mathbf{w}^T x_n - \mathbf{b}) \geq 1 - \xi_n \\ \xi_n \geq 0 \end{cases}, \quad n = 1, \dots, N \qquad (8.9)$$

where L represents the error penalty and e a vector of ones of N-dimension. Therefore, the optimization turns to a trade-off between a small error penalty and a large margin.

Table 8.5 details a new command, "fitcsvm," which can perform basic SVM training.

Fig. 8.4 Diagram of an SVM

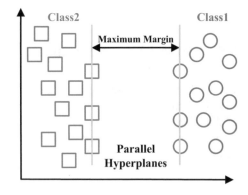

Table 8.5 The "fitcsvm" command

Mdl = fitcsvm(X,Y)
Input
X: predictor data
Y: class labels
Output
Mdl: trained SVM model

8.5.1 Generalized Eigenvalue Proximal Support Vector Machine

In the original SVM, two parallel planes are generated such that each plane is closest to one of the data sets and the two planes are as far apart as possible. Mangasarian and Wild [12] proposed the generalized eigenvalue proximal SVM (GEPSVM). It drops the parallelism condition on the two hyperplanes (remember that parallelism is necessary in the original SVM), and requires each hyperplane be as close as possible to one of the data sets, and as far away as possible from the other data set. The latest literature shows that GEPSVM achieved superior classification performance to canonical support vector machines.

Suppose samples are from either class 1 (denote by symbol X_1) or class 2 (denoted by symbol X_2). The GEPSVM finds the two optimal nonparallel planes [13] with the form:

$$\mathbf{w}_1^T x - \mathbf{b}_1 = 0 \text{ and } \mathbf{w}_2^T x - \mathbf{b}_2 = 0 \tag{8.10}$$

To obtain the first plane, we deduce from Eq. (8.10) and get the following solution:

$$(\mathbf{w}_1, \mathbf{b}_1) = \underset{(\mathbf{w},b)\neq 0}{\arg\min} \frac{\left\| \mathbf{w}^T X_1 - o^T \mathbf{b} \right\|^2 / \|z\|^2}{\left\| \mathbf{w}^T X_2 - o^T \mathbf{b} \right\|^2 / \|z\|^2} \tag{8.11}$$

$$z \leftarrow \begin{bmatrix} \mathbf{w} \\ \mathbf{b} \end{bmatrix} \tag{8.12}$$

where o is a vector of ones of appropriate dimensions. Simplifying Eq. (8.11) gives:

$$\underset{(\mathbf{w},b)\neq 0}{\min} \frac{\left\| \mathbf{w}^T X_1 - o^T b \right\|^2}{\left\| \mathbf{w}^T X_2 - o^T b \right\|^2} \tag{8.13}$$

We include the Tikhonov regularization term to decrease the norm of the variable z that corresponds to the first hyperplane in Eq. (8.10):

$$\min_{(\mathbf{w},b)\neq 0} \frac{\|\mathbf{w}^T X_1 - o^T b\|^2 + t\|z\|^2}{\|\mathbf{w}^T X_2 - o^T b\|^2} \tag{8.14}$$

where t is a positive (or zero) Tikhonov factor. Equation (8.14) turns to the "Rayleigh Quotient (RQ)" in the following form of:

$$z_1 = \arg\min_{z\neq 0} \frac{z^T P z}{z^T Q z} \tag{8.15}$$

where P and Q are symmetric matrices in $\mathbb{R}^{(p+1)\times(p+1)}$ as:

$$P \stackrel{\text{def}}{=} [X_1 \quad -o]^T [X_1 \quad -o] + tI \tag{8.16}$$

$$Q \stackrel{\text{def}}{=} [X_2 \quad -o]^T [X_2 \quad -o] \tag{8.17}$$

Using the stationarity and boundedness properties of the RQ, solution of Eq. (8.15) is deduced by solving a generalized eigenvalue problem as:

$$Pz = \lambda Q z, z \neq 0 \tag{8.18}$$

here the global minimum of Eq. (8.15) is obtained at an eigenvector z_1 corresponding to the smallest eigenvalue $\lambda_{\min}$ of Equaion (8.18). Therefore, $\mathbf{w}_1$ and b_1 can be obtained through Eq. (8.12), and used to determine the plane in Eq. (8.10). Afterwards, a similar optimization problem is generated that is analogous to Eq. (8.14) by exchanging the symbols of X_1 and X_2. The eigenvector z_2^* corresponding to the smallest eigenvalue of the second generalized eigenvalue problem will obtain the second hyperplane approximate to samples of class 2.

8.5.2 Twin Support Vector Machine

Jayadeva et al. [14] proposed a novel twin support vector machine (TSVM). It is similar to the GEPSVM in the way that both obtain non-parallel hyperplanes [15].

The difference lies in that the GEPSVM and TSVM are formulated entirely differently. Each of the two quadratic-programming (QP) problems in the TSVM pair is formulated as a typical SVM. Note that QP is a particular optimization problem in mathematics. It optimizes a quadratic function of several variables subject to linear constraints. Many mature approaches have been developed to solve QP problems, such as interior point, conjugate gradient, active set, augmented Lagrangian, and simplex algorithms.

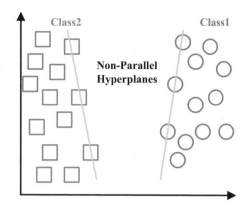

Fig. 8.5 Diagram of an NPSVM

Mathematically, the TSVM is constructed by solving the two QP problems:

$$\min_{\mathbf{w}_1,b_1,q} \frac{1}{2}\left(X_1\mathbf{w}_1 + o_1b_1\right)^{\mathrm{T}}\left(X_1\mathbf{w}_1 + o_1b_1\right) + c_1o_2^Tq$$
$$\text{s.t.} - \left(X_2\mathbf{w}_1 + o_2b_1\right) + q \geq o_2, q \geq 0 \tag{8.19}$$

$$\min_{\mathbf{w}_2,b_2,q} \frac{1}{2}\left(X_2\mathbf{w}_2 + o_2b_2\right)^{\mathrm{T}}\left(X_2\mathbf{w}_2 + o_2b_2\right) + c_2o_1^Tq$$
$$\text{s.t.} - \left(X_1\mathbf{w}_2 + o_1b_2\right) + q \geq o_1, q \geq 0 \tag{8.20}$$

here c_i ($i = 1, 2$) are positive parameters and o_i ($i = 1, 2$) is the same as in Eq. (8.11). By this means, the TSVM constructs two hyperplanes [16]. The first term in Eqs. (8.19) and (8.20) is the sum of squared distances from the hyperplane to one class. The second term is the sum of error variables. Therefore, minimizing Eqs. (8.19) and (8.20) will keep the hyperplanes close to points of each class, and minimize the misclassification rate. Finally, the constraint requires the hyperplane to be at a distance of more than one from points of the other class. Another advantage of the TSVM is that its convergence rate is four times faster than conventional SVMs.

Both the GEPSVM and TSVM are termed as non-parallel SVMs (NPSVMs) [17], a diagram of which shown in Fig. 8.5. Compared to the standard SVM in Fig. 8.4, the NPSVM discards parallelism, and so is more flexible than the SVM.

8.5.3 Fuzzy Support Vector Machines

A fuzzy SVM (FSVM) is more effective than simple SVM models especially in predicting or classifying real-world data, because several training samples are more substantial than others. It makes sense to require that the meaningful training samples must be recognized perfectly meanwhile to neglect some meaningless points like noise or outliers.

FSVM apply a fuzzy membership function (FMF) s to every training point, such that the training samples are transferred to fuzzy training samples, which can be expressed as:

$$\{(x_n, y_n, s_n)|x_n \in \mathbb{R}^z, 0 < s_n \leq 1\}, n = 1, \ldots, N \tag{8.21}$$

where s_n denotes the altitude of the corresponding training point toward one class and $(1-s_n)$ is the attitude of meaning less. The optimal hyperplane problem of a FSVM is defined as:

$$\min_{\mathbf{w},\xi,\mathbf{b}} \frac{1}{2}\|\mathbf{w}\|^2 + c\mathbf{s}^T\boldsymbol{\xi}$$
$$s.t. \begin{cases} y_n(\mathbf{w}^T x_n - \mathbf{b}) \geq 1 - \xi_n \\ \xi_n \geq 0 \end{cases}, n = 1, \ldots, N \tag{8.22}$$

where $\mathbf{s} = (s_1, s_2, \ldots, s_N)$ represents the membership vector of the FMF. A smaller s_n decreases the influence of the parameter ξ_n, such that the corresponding sample p_n is regarded less substantial [18].

8.6 Multiclass Technique

The SVM was originally designed for binary classification problems. Several methods were proposed for multiclass problems, and the dominant multiclass technique was to reduce the single multiclass problem into multiple binary classification problems.

8.6.1 Winner-Take-All

Assume there are totally C (>2) classes. The winner-take-all (WTA) strategy classifies new instances based on the idea of one-versus-all. We first train C different binary classifiers (e.g., the SVMs), each one trained to distinguish the data in a single class from the data of all the remaining classes. When applied to new test data, all the C classifiers are run, and the classifier that outputs the largest value is chosen [19]. If there are two identical output values, WTA selects the class with the smallest index.

The mathematical model is described as follow. Given an A-dimensional, N-size training data set of the form:

$$\{(x_n, y_n) | x_n \in \mathbb{R}^A, y_n \in \{1, 2, \ldots, C\}\}, n = 1, 2, \ldots, N \qquad (8.23)$$

where x_n is an A-dimensional vector and y_n is the known class label of each x_n. The classification score S for the cth individual binary classifier can be defined as:

$$S_c(x) = \sum_{n=1}^{N} y_n^c \alpha_n^c k(x_n, x) - b_c, \ c = 1, 2, \ldots, C \qquad (8.24)$$

with the interpreted output as:

$$y_n^c = \begin{cases} +1 & \text{if } x_n \in c\text{th class} \\ -1 & \text{otherwise} \end{cases} \qquad (8.25)$$

where c represents the class index; S the score; N the number of training data; $y_n^c \in \{+1, -1\}$ depends on the class label of x_n, if x_n belongs to the cth class, $y_n^c = +1$, otherwise $y_n^c = -1$; $k(\ )$ is the predefined kernel function; α_n^c is the Lagrange coefficient; and b_c is the bias term. α_n^c and b_c are obtained by training the cth individual binary classifier. The final output of the whole classifier is:

$$o(x) = \arg\max_{c \in C} S_c(x) \qquad (8.26)$$

Here we use the "argmax" function instead of the "sign" function that is commonly used in binary classification. Figure 8.6 gives an illustration of this. Suppose we had four different classes and therefore established four individual classifiers. The first classifier "1v1" means that all the samples in class 1 are positive and all samples outside class 1 are negative. The scores of the four classifiers are:

- $S_1(x) = -0.9$.
- $S_2(x) = -0.7$.
- $S_3(x) = 0.5$.
- $S_4(x) = 0.3$.

Fig. 8.6 Diagram of WTA

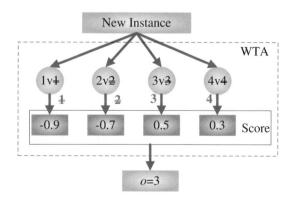

The third classifier is selected because its score was the largest among all individual classifiers, and the given instance was recognized as class 3.

8.6.2   Max-Wins-Voting

The max-wins-voting (MWV) classifies a new instance based on the one-versus-one approach. We construct a binary individual classifier for each pair of classes, so in total we will get $C(C - 1)/2$ individual binary classifiers. When applied to new test data, each individual classifier gives one vote to the winning class, and the test data is labeled with the class having most votes. If there are two identical votes, MWV selects the class with the smallest index.

The mathematical model is described as follows. The ij-th ($i = 1,2, ..., C - 1$, $j = i + 1, ..., C$) individual binary classifier is trained with all data in the ith class with a $+1$ label and all data of the jth class with a -1 label, so as to distinguish the ith class from jth class. The classification score of the ij-th individual classifier is:

$$S_{ij}(x) = \sum_{n=1}^{N_i + N_j} y_n^{ij} \alpha_n^{ij} k(x_n^{ij}, x) - b_{ij}$$

$$i = 1, 2, \ldots, C - 1, j = i + 1, i + 2, \ldots, C \tag{8.27}$$

The interpretation output result is:

$$y_n^{ij} = \begin{cases} +1 & x_n^{ij} \in i\text{th class} \\ -1 & x_n^{ij} \in j\text{th class} \end{cases} \tag{8.28}$$

where N_i and N_j denote the total number of ith class and jth class, respectively; $y_n^{ij} \in \{+1, -1\}$ depends on the class label of x_n^{ij}, if x_n^{ij} belongs to ith class, $y_n^{ij} = +1$, otherwise x_n^{ij} belongs to jth class, $y_n^{ij} = -1$; α_n^{ij} is the Lagrange coefficient; and b_{ij} is the bias term. α_n^{ij} and b_{ij} are obtained by training the ij-th individual SVM. The output of the ij-th individual classifier is the sign function of its score, namely:

$$o_{ij}(x) = \text{sgn}(S_{ij}(x)) \tag{8.29}$$

If $S_{ij}(x) > 0$, then the output $o_{ij}(x)$ is $+1$, denoting that x belongs to the ith class; otherwise the output is -1, denoting x belongs to the jth class. The final output of the MWV is:

$$o(x) = \arg\max_i \left(\sum_j o_{ij}(x) \right) \tag{8.30}$$

Fig. 8.7 Diagram of MWV

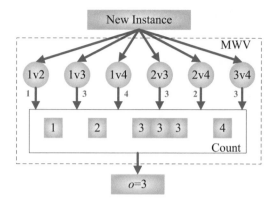

Figure 8.7 shows MWV. There are four classes in total, so six classifiers are established. For the new instance:

- Individual classifier 1 outputs 1.
- Individual classifier 2 outputs 3.
- Individual classifier 3 outputs 4.
- Individual classifier 4 outputs 3.
- Individual classifier 5 outputs 2.
- Individual classifier 6 outputs 3.

We do a count of the results and note that there are 3 classifiers that output 3, and only 1 classifier that outputs 1, 2, and 4. Therefore, class 3 is the final choice.

8.6.3   Directed Acyclic Graph

The directed acyclic graph (DAG) is a graph whose edges have an orientation and no cycles. The whole classifier constructs the same individual classifier set as the MWV using a one-versus-one model, however, the output of each individual classifier is explained differently. When $o_{ij}(x)$ is +1, it denotes that x does not belong to jth class; when $o_{ij}(x)$ is −1, it denotes that x does not belong to ith class. Therefore, the final decision cannot be reached, until the leaf node is reached.

Figure 8.8 shows the DAG for finding the optimal class out of 4 classes. Here, the root node and intermediate nodes represent the individual binary classifier, whereas the leaf nodes represent the output label [20]. Given a test sample x starting at the root node, the individual binary classifiers are evaluated. The node is then exited via the evaluation result to either left edge or right edge [21]. The next individual classifier's function is evaluated again until the leaf node is reached. Therefore, the whole classifier generated by a DAG uses less computation time compared to one generated by MWV.

Fig. 8.8 Diagram of a DAG

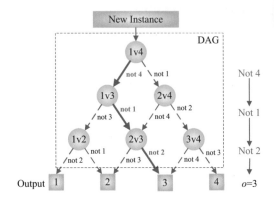

8.7   Feed-Forward Neural Network

The feed-forward neural network (FNN) belongs to one type of artificial neural network. It is different from recurrent neural networks [22], since the connections within the FNN do not form a cycle. The FNN is also called the multilayer perceptron (MLP). In this book, we focus on the single-hidden-layer FNN. Its structure is shown in Fig. 8.9.

Table 8.6 details Matlab's "feedforwardnet" command, which can establish an FNN with a given number of hidden neurons and training functions. Table 8.7 details "patternnet," another command which can be used to adjust the performance function.

8.7.1   Encoding Strategy

Let N_I represent the number of input neurons, N_H the number of hidden neurons, and N_O the number of output neurons. Suppose ω_1 and ω_2 represent the connection weight matrix between the input layer and hidden layer, and between the hidden layer and the output layer, respectively.

Figure 8.10 details the formation of the weight matrix (ω_1, ω_2). The encoding style can be presented as the combination of the vectorization of (ω_1, ω_2):

$$
\omega = [\mathcal{V}(\omega_1), \mathcal{V}(\omega_2)]
$$
$$
= \left[\underbrace{\omega_1(1,1), \ldots \omega_1(N_I, N_H)}_{N_I * N_H}, \underbrace{\omega_2(1,1), \ldots \omega_2(N_H, N_O)}_{N_H * N_O} \right] \tag{8.31}
$$

where $\mathcal{V}$ represents the vectorization operation.

Fig. 8.9 Structure of the single-hidden-layer FNN

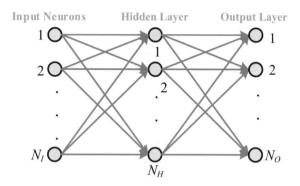

Table 8.6 The "feedforwardnet" command	**net = feedforwardnet(hs, trainFcn)**
	Input hs: size of hidden layer trainFcn: training function
	Output net: established net

Table 8.7 The "patternnet" command	**net = patternnet (hs, trainFcn, performFcn)**
	Input hs: size of hidden layer trainFcn: training function performFcn: performance function[a]
	Output net: established net

[a]Default is the cross-entropy criterion

8.7.2   Criterion

Subsequently, we can infer the criterion of a single-hidden-layer FNN, i.e., the training process to update these weighted values, which can be divided into four steps:

(1) The outputs of all neurons in the hidden layer are calculated by:

$$y_j = f_H \left(\sum_{i=1}^{N_I} \omega_1(i,j) x_i \right) j = 1, 2, \cdots, N_H \tag{8.32}$$

Here x_i denotes the ith input value; y_j denotes the jth output of the hidden layer; and f_H is referred to as the activation function (AF) of the hidden layer.

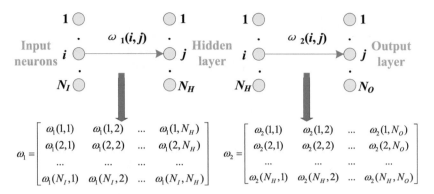

Fig. 8.10 The connection weight matrices

(2) The outputs of all neurons in the output layer are given as follows:

$$O_k = f_O \left(\sum_{j=1}^{N_H} \omega_2(j,k)y_j \right) k = 1, 2, \ldots, N_O \qquad (8.33)$$

Here f_O denotes the activation function of output layer. All weights are assigned with random values initially, and are modified traditionally by the delta rule according to the learning samples.

(3) The error is expressed as the mean squared error (MSE) [23] of the difference between the output and target value:

$$E_l = \mathrm{mse} \left(\sum_{k=1}^{N_O} (O_k - T_k) \right) l = 1, 2, \ldots N_S \qquad (8.33)$$

where T_k represents the kth value of the authentic values which are already known to users and N_S represents the number of samples.

(4) The criterion is usually written as the average MSE:

$$f(\omega) = \sum_{l=1}^{N_S} E_l \qquad (8.34)$$

The goal is to minimize this fitness function $f(\omega)$, viz., force the output values of each sample to approximate to corresponding target values.

In a word, the weights of an FNN are regarded as the variables, and average MSE between the output and target is regarded as the criterion. The weights optimization problem is finding the best weights to minimize the average MSE.

8.7.3 Activation Function

In neuroscience, activation function s (AFs) represent the rate of action potential firing the cell. Its simplest form is binary, viz., either firing or not firing. For the SLFN, we need to discuss the AF in output units and hidden units separately [24].

In terms of the activation function f_O of the output layer, there are normally three types: (1) the linear function for the Gaussian output distribution, (2) the logistic sigmoid function [25] for the Bernoulli output distribution, and (3) the softmax function [26] for the Multinoulli output distribution.

The logistic sigmoid (LOSI) function is defined as:

$$f_O(x) = \frac{1}{1 + \exp(-x)} \tag{8.35}$$

Determining the AF f_H of the hidden units is more problematic. Traditionally, the LOSI function has been used as the AF of hidden units. More recently, scholars have pointed out that the widespread saturation of the sigmoidal function makes gradient-based learning very difficult. Hence, the rectified linear unit (ReLU) [27] was proposed since it is more biologically plausible, and ReLUs were used to act as the AF for hidden units, with the following formula:

$$\text{ReLU} : f_H(x) = \max(0, x) \tag{8.36}$$

Nevertheless, the ReLU cannot learn via gradient-based methods when activation values are zero. Hence, a leaky ReLU (LReLU) is used, which allows a small gradient when the unit is not active:

$$\text{LReLU} : f_H(x) = \begin{cases} x & x > 0 \\ 0.01x & \text{otherwise} \end{cases} \tag{8.37}$$

We can compare the three AFs above. Their curves are shown in Fig. 8.11.

8.8 Extreme Learning Machines

An extreme learning machine (ELM) is a learning method that is used to train the single-hidden-layer neural network [28]. An ELM can solve regression and classification problems. One of the most important characteristics of an ELM is that it converges much faster than conventional learning algorithms, and matches them in terms of performance.

Fig. 8.11 AFs: **a** LOSI;
b ReLU; **c** LReLU

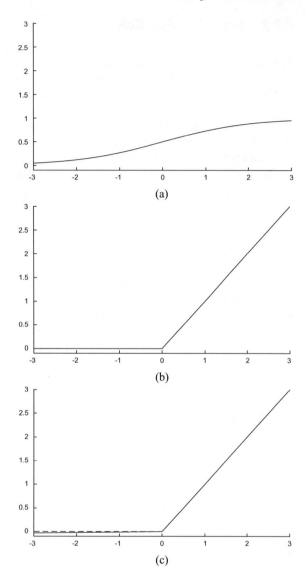

(a)

(b)

(c)

8.8.1   Structure

There are three layers in an ELM, as shown in Fig. 8.12. The neurons in adjacent layers are fully linked. The weights and biases from the input layer to the hidden layer are randomly assigned [29], and the biases from the hidden layer to the output layer are also set randomly. It is required that the AF in the hidden layer be infinitely differentiable. The only parameter that needs to be trained is the weight matrix that links hidden and output neurons [30].

Fig. 8.12 Structure of an
ELM

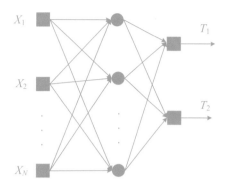

Table 8.8 Pseudocode of an
ELM

Step1: Assign input weight W_i and bias b_i at random
Step2: Compute the output matrix H of hidden layer
Step3: Obtain the output weight $\boldsymbol{\beta} = \boldsymbol{H}^{+}\boldsymbol{T}$, where $T = [t_1, t_2, \ldots, t_N]^{\text{T}}$, and H^{+} represents the Moore–Penrose generalized inverse of H

In general, the algorithm is expressed as follows: for a training set $X = [(x_i, t_i)|$ $i = 1,2,\ldots, N]$, suppose the hidden node number is N and then apply the pseudocode in Table 8.8.

8.8.2 Online Sequential Extreme Learning Machine

Liang et al. [31] proposed a variant of the ELM—the online sequential extreme learning machine (OSELM). Unlike the common ELM, which is trained in batch mode, OSELM is implemented in online sequential mode [32]. This means the OSELM does not need to be re-trained when new data is received [33], which satisfies some online industrial applications. Given an AF f, and hidden neuron number $\hat{N}$, the training algorithm consists of two phases as follows.

Phase I. For a small initial training dataset:

$$S = \{(x_i, y_i)|x_i \in R^n, y_i \in R^m, i = 1, \ldots, N\} \tag{8.38}$$

1. Randomly assign the weight from input to hidden layer W_i and the hidden layer bias b_i.
2. Compute the initial output matrix of the hidden layer:

$$H_0 = [h_1, \ldots, h_{\widehat{N}}]^{\text{T}} \tag{8.39}$$

where

$$h_i = [f(w_1 x_i + b_1), \ldots, f(w_{\widehat{N}} x_i + b_{\widehat{N})}]^T, i = 1, \ldots, \widehat{N} \tag{8.40}$$

3. Calculate the output weight:

$$\beta_0 = M_0 H_0^T T_0 \tag{8.41}$$

where

$$M_0 = (H_0^T H_0)^{-1} \tag{8.42}$$

$$T_0 = [t_1, \ldots, t_{\widehat{N}}]^T \tag{8.43}$$

4. Set $t = 0$.

Phase II. For each new sample (x_i, y_i), where $x_i \in R^n$, $y_i \in R^m$, and $i = \widehat{N} + 1, \widehat{N} + 2, \widehat{N} + 3, \ldots$

1. Estimate the hidden layer output:

$$h_{(t+1)} = [f(w_1 x_i + b_1), \ldots, f(w_{\widehat{N}} x_i + b_{\widehat{N}})]^T \tag{8.44}$$

2. Modify the weight from the hidden layer to the output layer $\beta_{(t+1)}$ using the recursive least-square algorithm:

$$M_{t+1} = M_t - \frac{M_t h_{t+1} h_{t+1}^T M_t}{1 + h_{t+1}^T M_t h_{t+1}} \tag{8.45}$$

$$\beta_{(t+1)} = \beta_{(t)} + M_{t+1} h_{t+1} (t_i^T - h_{t+1}^T \beta_{(t)}) \tag{8.46}$$

3. Set $k = k + 1$.

Several other important variants of the ELM exist: evolutionary ELM (EELM), incremental ELM (IELM), optimally pruned ELM (OPELM), etc.

8.8.3 Controversy

The ELM has raised some controversy since 2008. Wang and Wan [34] pointed out that the essence of the ELM appeared earlier in work by Broomhead et al. They believed it was not necessary to introduce a new name for the "ELM." The machine-learning expert Yann LeCun also queried "What's so great about ELMs?"

8.9 Radial Basis Function Neural Network

A radial basis function neural network (RBFNN) is a FNN that uses radial basis function as its AFs [35].

8.9.1 Structure

An RBFNN has three main features: a universal approximator, best-approximation property, and optimality [36]. As is illustrated in Fig. 8.13, an RBFNN usually consists of an input layer, a hidden layer, and an output layer. An M-dimensional vector serves as the input layer [37], which is fully connected with the hidden layer consisting of N neurons. The hidden layer neurons are fully linked to the output layer, which is made up of J neurons.

The Gaussian RBFNN is the most often used—it is determined by mean vectors m_i and covariance matrixes C_i, $i = 1, 2, \ldots, N$. In simple terms, the activation function of the ith hidden neuron for an input vector x_m is as follows:

$$g_i(x_m) = \exp\left(\frac{-||x_m - m_i||}{2\sigma_i^2}\right) \tag{8.47}$$

where σ_i^2 and m_i can be calculated using a clustering algorithm. The number of AFs and values of spread parameters characterize the smoothness of the mapping.

The weights ω_{ij} connects the hidden units to output units. Here we give the jth output for an input x_m:

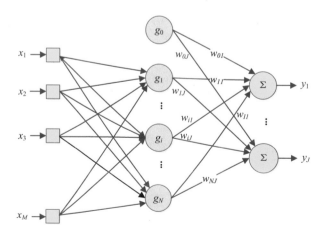

Fig. 8.13 Structure of an RBFNN

$$y_j(x_m) = \sum_{i=0}^{N} \omega_{ij} g_i(x_m), j = 1, 2, \ldots, J \qquad (8.48)$$

where

$$g_0(x_m) = 1 \qquad (8.49)$$

8.9.2 Training

Training the RBFNN can be divided into two stages:

- Establishing basis functions.
- Fixing the weights from the hidden nodes to the output neurons.

For the first stage, we employ k-means clustering which sorts all the objects into a defined number of groups in order to minimize the total squared Euclidian distance for each object and consider its nearest cluster center at the same time.

For the second stage, we calculate the weights easily by matrix inversion and matrix multiplication, since the AFs of output neurons are linear.

Two commands can be used to design an RBFNN: "newrb" and "newrbe." Their input and output arguments are detailed in Tables 8.9 and 8.10, respectively.

Table 8.9 The "newrb" command

net = newrb(P, T, goal, spread, MN, DF)
Input
P: input vectors
T: target class vectors
goal: MSE goal
spread: spread of RBF
MN: maximum number of neurons
DF: number of neurons to add between displays
Output
net: an established RBFNNt

Table 8.10 The "newrbe" command

net = newrbe(P, T, spread)
Input
P: input vectors
T: target class vectors
spread: spread of RBF
Output
net: an established RBFNN

8.10 Probabilistic Neural Network

The probabilistic neural network (PNN) has gained interest in recent years, as it yields a probabilistic score for each input.

Suppose there are two classes (A and B), we should decide which class the sample $x = [x_1, \ldots, x_N]$ belongs to. Suppose h_A and h_B represent the a priori probability of instances in class A and B, respectively, the Bayes' decision rule turns to:

$$\text{Class}(x) = \begin{cases} A & \text{if } l_A h_A f_A(x) > l_B h_B f_B(x) \\ B & \text{otherwise} \end{cases} \tag{8.50}$$

where l_A represents the loss function of the wrong decision that x is in class B when class(x) = A, and the same for l_B. The losses are equal to zero for correct corrections [38]. f_A and f_B are the probability density function (PDF) of classes A and B, respectively [39].

In a simple case that the $l_A = l_B$ and $h_A = h_B$, the classifier predicts a new instance to the class with a higher PDF [40]. To embed the Gaussian kernel, the PDF of class A can be expressed as:

$$f_A(x) = \frac{1}{(2\pi)^{N/2} \sigma^N} \frac{1}{T_A} \sum_{j=1}^{T_A} \exp\left[-\frac{(x - x_{Aj})^T (x - x_{Aj})}{2s^2} \right] \tag{8.51}$$

Here, s is the smoothing factor; T_A the number of training samples in class A; and x_{Aj} the jth sample in class A.

Figure 8.14 illustrates the structure of a PNN. Its mathematical expressions are:

$$a = f_r(b * \|I - x\|) \tag{8.52}$$

$$y = f_c(a * L) \tag{8.53}$$

where I denotes input weight; L the layer weight; f_r the radial basis function; and f_c the compete function:

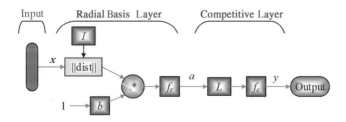

Fig. 8.14 Structure of a PNN

Table 8.11 The "newpnn" command	**net = newpnn(P, T, spread)**
	Input P: input vectors T: target class vectors spread: spread of RBF
	Output net: an established PNN

$$f_r(x) = \exp(-x^2)$$
$$f_c(x) = e_x = [0\ldots0\ \underset{x}{1}\ 0\ldots0] \tag{8.54}$$

Table 8.11 details Matlab's "newpnn" command which can help when designing a PNN.

8.11 Linear Regression Classifier

The linear regression–based classification method utilizes linear regression to measure the distance from a sample to a specific class. Suppose the samples from the same class lie on a linear subspace. We can represent a sample by the linear combinations of its intra-class sample, where linear regression is used to calculate the reconstruction error (the distance from a sample to a specific class).

For a sample from an unknown class, we employ samples from each class to compute the reconstruction error. The label of the sample will be assigned as the class with the smallest reconstruction error.

The linear regression classifier (LRC) is a classical classification method. Assume there is a data set $X = [X_1, X_2,\ldots, X_m]$. Here m represents the number of classes. Suppose samples from a specific class lie on a linear subspace. A brain image t_i from the ith class can be expressed as a combination of the samples from the same class X_i:

$$t_i = X_i d_i \tag{8.55}$$

where d_i is the reconstruction coefficient which can be calculated from the least-squares estimation (LSE) [41]:

$$\hat{d}_i = \left(X_i^T X_i\right)^{-1} X_i^T t_i \tag{8.56}$$

Then the brain image t_i is reconstructed as:

$$\hat{t}_i = X_i \hat{d}_i \tag{8.57}$$

The reconstruction error r_i of the ith class is used to estimate the similarity between the brain image and the ith class, which is defined as follows:

$$r_i = t_i - \hat{t}_i = t_i - X_i \hat{d}_i \tag{8.58}$$

For an unknown brain image p, we can employ all the m class models to compute the reconstruction error. Finally, the label of the test brain image p is assigned as:

$$\text{label}(p) = \min_i \left\| p - X_i \hat{d}_i \right\|^2 \tag{8.59}$$

8.12 Conclusion

In this Chapter, we compared several important classifiers. There are many other popular classifiers, such as logistic regression, convolution neural network, shared-weight neural network, etc. Readers are encouraged to test these advanced classifiers during future studies.

References

1. Torgo L, Branco P, Ribeiro RP, Pfahringer B (2015) Resampling strategies for regression. Expert Syst 32(3):465–476. https://doi.org/10.1111/exsy.12081
2. Punitha K, Latha B (2016) Sampling imbalance dataset for software defect prediction using hybrid neuro-fuzzy systems with naive bayes classifier. Tehnicki Vjesnik-Tech Gaz 23 (6):1795–1804. https://doi.org/10.17559/tv-20151219112129
3. Swetapadma A, Yadav A (2016) Protection of parallel transmission lines including inter-circuit faults using Naive Bayes classifier. Alexandria Eng J 55(2):1411–1419. https://doi.org/10.1016/j.aej.2016.03.029
4. Rahmatian M, Chen YC, Palizban A, Moshref A, Dunford WG (2017) Transient stability assessment via decision trees and multivariate adaptive regression splines. Electr Power Syst Res 142:320–328. https://doi.org/10.1016/j.epsr.2016.09.030
5. Sathyadevan S, Nair RR (2015) Comparative analysis of decision tree algorithms: ID3, C4.5 and random forest. In: Jain LC, Behera HS, Mandal JK, Mohapatra DP (eds) Computational intelligence in data mining. Smart innovation systems and technologies, vol 31. Springer, Berlin, pp 549–562. https://doi.org/10.1007/978-81-322-2205-7_51
6. Zimmerman RK, Balasubramani GK, Nowalk MP, Eng H, Urbanski L, Jackson ML, Jackson LA, McLean HQ, Belongia EA, Monto AS, Malosh RE, Gaglani M, Clipper L, Flannery B, Wisniewski SR (2016) Classification and regression tree (CART) analysis to predict influenza in primary care patients. BMC Infect Dis 16, Article ID: 503. https://doi.org/10.1186/s12879-016-1839-x

7. Youssef AM, Pourghasemi HR, Pourtaghi ZS, Al-Katheeri MM (2016) Landslide susceptibility mapping using random forest, boosted regression tree, classification and regression
tree, and general linear models and comparison of their performance at Wadi Tayyah Basin,
Asir Region, Saudi Arabia. Landslides 13(5):839–856. https://doi.org/10.1007/s10346-015-
0614-1

8. McRoberts RE, Domke GM, Chen Q, Naesset E, Gobakken T (2016) Using genetic
algorithms to optimize k-Nearest neighbors configurations for use with airborne laser
scanning data. Remote Sens Environ 184:387–395. https://doi.org/10.1016/j.rse.2016.07.007

9. Amiri M, Amnieh HB, Hasanipanah M, Khanli LM (2016) A new combination of artificial
neural network and K-nearest neighbors models to predict blast-induced ground vibration and
air-overpressure. Eng Comput 32(4):631–644. https://doi.org/10.1007/s00366-016-0442-5

10. Chon AT (2010) Design of Lazy Classifier based on Fuzzy k-Nearest Neighbors and
Reconstruction Error (퍼지 k-Nearest Neighbors 와 Reconstruction Error 기반 Lazy
Classifier 설계). J Korean Inst Intell Syst 20(1):101–108

11. Zhang LA, Parker RS, Swigon D, Banerjee I, Bahrami S, Redl H, Clermont G (2016) A
one-nearest-neighbor approach to identify the original time of infection using censored
baboon sepsis data. Crit Care Med 44(6):E432–E442. https://doi.org/10.1097/ccm.
0000000000001623

12. Mangasarian OL, Wild EW (2006) Multisurface proximal support vector machine classification via generalized eigenvalues. IEEE Trans Pattern Anal Mach Intell 28(1):69–74. https://
doi.org/10.1109/tpami.2006.17

13. Yang J (2015) Preclinical diagnosis of magnetic resonance (MR) brain images via discrete
wavelet packet transform with Tsallis entropy and generalized eigenvalue proximal support
vector machine (GEPSVM). Entropy 17(4):1795–1813. https://doi.org/10.3390/e17041795

14. Jayadeva, Khemchandani R., Chandra S. (2007) Twin support vector machines for pattern
classification. IEEE Trans Pattern Anal Mach Intell 29(5):905–910. https://doi.org/10.1109/
tpami.2007.1068

15. Yang M (2016) Dual-tree complex wavelet transform and twin support vector machine for
pathological brain detection. Appl Sci 6(6), Article ID: 169

16. Yadav AK, Mehta R, Kumar R, Vishwakarma VP (2016) Lagrangian twin support vector
regression and genetic algorithm based robust grayscale image watermarking. Multimedia
Tools Appl 75(15):9371–9394. https://doi.org/10.1007/s11042-016-3381-7

17. Chen S, Yang J-F, Phillips P (2015) Magnetic resonance brain image classification based on
weighted-type fractional Fourier transform and nonparallel support vector machine. Int J
Imaging Syst Technol 25(4):317–327. https://doi.org/10.1002/ima.22144

18. Lu HM (2016) Facial emotion recognition based on biorthogonal wavelet entropy, fuzzy
support vector machine, and stratified cross validation. IEEE Access 4:8375–8385. https://doi.
org/10.1109/ACCESS.2016.2628407

19. Kuri-Morales A, Mejia-Guevara I (2006) Evolutionary training of SVM for multiple category
classification problems with self-adaptive parameters. In: Sichman JS, Coelho H, Rezende SO
(eds) 10th Ibero-American conference on artificial intelligence/18th Brazilian symposium on
artificial intelligence, Riberiao Preto, Brazil. Lecture Notes in computer science. Springer,
pp 329–338

20. Cholissodin I, Kurniawati M, Indriati, Arwani I (2014) Classification of campus e-complaint
documents using directed acyclic graph multi-class SVM based on analytic hierarchy process.
In: International conference on advanced computer science and information system, Jakarta,
Indonesia. IEEE, pp 247–253. https://doi.org/10.1109/icacsis.2014.7065835

21. Gorriz JM, Ramírez J (2016) Wavelet entropy and directed acyclic graph support vector
machine for detection of patients with unilateral hearing loss in MRI scanning. Front Comput
Neurosci 10, Article ID: 160. https://doi.org/10.3389/fncom.2016.00106

22. King RTFA, Tu X, Dessaint LA, Kamwa I (2016) Multi-contingency transient
stability-constrained optimal power flow using multilayer feedforward neural networks. In:
Canadian conference on electrical and computer engineering (CCECE), Canada. IEEE, pp 1–
6. https://doi.org/10.1109/ccece.2016.7726774

23. Dolezel P, Skrabanek P, Gago L (2016) Detection of grapes in natural environment using feedforward neural network as a classifier. In: SAI computing conference, London, UK. IEEE, pp 1330–1334. https://doi.org/10.1109/sai.2016.7556153

24. Njikam ANS, Zhao H (2016) A novel activation function for multilayer feed-forward neural networks. Appl Intell 45(1):75–82. https://doi.org/10.1007/s10489-015-0744-0

25. Zadeh MR, Amin S, Khalili D, Singh VP (2010) Daily outflow prediction by multi layer perceptron with logistic sigmoid and tangent sigmoid activation functions. Water Resour Manage 24(11):2673–2688. https://doi.org/10.1007/s11269-009-9573-4

26. Liao B, Xu JG, Lv JT, Zhou SL (2015) An image retrieval method for binary images based on DBN and softmax classifier. IETE Tech Rev 32(4):294–303. https://doi.org/10.1080/02564602.2015.1015631

27. Hara K, Saito D, Shouno H (2015) Analysis of function of rectified linear unit used in deep learning. In: International joint conference on neural networks, Killarney, Ireland, IEEE international joint conference on neural networks (IJCNN). IEEE, pp 144–151

28. Al-Yaseen WL, Othman ZA, Nazri MZA (2017) Multi-level hybrid support vector machine and extreme learning machine based on modified K-means for intrusion detection system. Expert Syst Appl 67:296–303. https://doi.org/10.1016/j.eswa.2016.09.041

29. Sokolov-Mladenovic S, Milovancevic M, Mladenovic I, Alizamir M (2016) Economic growth forecasting by artificial neural network with extreme learning machine based on trade, import and export parameters. Comput Hum Behav 65:43–45. https://doi.org/10.1016/j.chb.2016.08.014

30. Sungheetha A, Sharma RR (2016) Extreme learning machine and fuzzy K-nearest neighbour based hybrid gene selection technique for cancer classification. J Med Imaging Health Inform 6(7):1652–1656. https://doi.org/10.1166/jmihi.2016.1866

31. Liang NY, Huang GB, Saratchandran P, Sundararajan N (2006) A fast and accurate online sequential learning algorithm for feedforward networks. IEEE Trans Neural Networks 17 (6):1411–1423. https://doi.org/10.1109/tnn.2006.880583

32. Meruane V (2016) Online sequential extreme learning machine for vibration-based damage assessment using transmissibility data. J Comput Civil Eng 30(3), Article ID: 04015042. https://doi.org/10.1061/(asce)cp.1943-5487.0000517

33. Ghimire D, Lee J (2016) Online sequential extreme learning machine-based co-training for dynamic moving cast shadow detection. Multimedia Tools Appl 75(18):11181–11197. https://doi.org/10.1007/s11042-015-2839-3

34. Wang LPP, Wan CRR (2008) Comments on "The Extreme Learning Machine.". IEEE Trans Neural Networks 19(8):1494–1495. https://doi.org/10.1109/tnn.2008.2002273

35. Li MN, Kwak KC, Kim YT (2016) Estimation of energy expenditure using a patch-type sensor module with an incremental radial basis function neural network. Sensors 16(10), Article ID: 1566. https://doi.org/10.3390/s16101566

36. Mateo-Sotos J, Torres AM, Sanchez-Morla EV, Santos JL (2016) An adaptive radial basis function neural network filter for noise reduction in biomedical recordings. Circ Syst Sig Process 35(12):4463–4485. https://doi.org/10.1007/s00034-016-0281-z

37. Lu Z (2016) A pathological brain detection system based on radial basis function neural network. J Med Imaging Health Inform 6(5):1218–1222

38. Nagamani G, Radhika T (2015) Dissipativity and passivity analysis of T-S fuzzy neural networks with probabilistic time-varying delays: a quadratic convex combination approach. Nonlinear Dyn 82(3):1325–1341. https://doi.org/10.1007/s11071-015-2241-8

39. Naggaz N, Wei G (2009) Remote-sensing image classification based on an improved probabilistic neural network. Sensors 9(9):7516–7539

40. Padil KH, Bakhary N, Hao H (2017) The use of a non-probabilistic artificial neural network to consider uncertainties in vibration-based-damage detection. Mech Syst Signal Process 83:194–209. https://doi.org/10.1016/j.ymssp.2016.06.007

41. Chen Y, Zhang Y, Lu H (2016) Wavelet energy entropy and linear regression classifier for detecting abnormal breasts. Multimedia Tools Appl. https://doi.org/10.1007/s11042-016-4161-0

Chapter 9
Weight Optimization of Classifiers for Pathological Brain Detection

This chapter gives the latest training methods for training the weights and biases of feed-forward neural networks (FNNs). Note that the training is not pure optimization; hence, the training should be over the validation set. The traditional back propagation scheme, performed by the gradient descent method, and its variants, are reviewed. Later, 10 global optimization methods are compared, including the genetic algorithm, simulate annealing, the tabu search, the artificial immune system, particle swarm optimization, artificial bee colony, the firefly algorithm, ant colony optimization, biogeography-based optimization, and the Jaya algorithm. The Jaya algorithm does not need to set common controlling parameters, and only needs to set population size and maximum iteration number. For each method, the idea that inspires the corresponding method is given. The mathematical equations and pipeline diagrams of these methods are provided and compared. In particular, the effect of optimization for pathological brain detection (PBD) is analyzed. The early stopping method is an essential subtlety, since training a classifier is not a pure optimization problem.

9.1 Backpropagation

9.1.1 Traditional Methods

There are many successful optimization methods, which can train the FNN. For example, the traditional backpropagation (BP) is usually in used in conjunction with the gradient descent method. It is composed of two phases as shown in Table 9.1. Other variants of BP include adaptive BP, momentum BP, etc.

Several commands in Matlab can be employed to help train neural networks, as shown in Table 9.2.

© Springer Nature Singapore Pte Ltd. 2018   149
S.-H. Wang et al., *Pathological Brain Detection*, Brain Informatics and Health,
https://doi.org/10.1007/978-981-10-4026-9_9

Table 9.1 Pseudocode of BP

Phase	Name	Implementation
I	Propagation	The training sample is forward propagated through the FNN, and the error is backward propagated
II	Weight update	The current weight is updated by subtracting from the gradient of the weight

Table 9.2 Matlab commands to train the FNN

Command	Aim
trainbfg	Broyden–Fletcher–Goldfarb–Shanno (BFGS) quasi-Newton BP
traincgb	Conjugate gradient BP with Powell–Beale restarts
traincgf	Conjugate gradient BP with Fletcher–Reeves updates
traincgp	Conjugate gradient BP with Polak–Ribiére updates
traindgm	Gradient descent with momentum BP
traingda	Gradient descent with adaptive learning rate BP
traingdx	Gradient descent with momentum and adaptive learning rate BP
trainlm	Levenberg–Marquardt BP
trainoss	One-step secant BP
trainrp	Resilient BP
trainscg	Scaled conjugate gradient BP

9.1.2   Shortcomings

Nevertheless, BP and its variants suffer from convergence which is too slow along with unreliable training. The algorithm may become trapped in local minima other than global minima (Fig. 9.1), thus, metaheuristic methods are usually employed to train the weight.

It is unnecessary to use part of the whole data set to reduce training time, which is routine in deep learning. The reason for this is the small size data sets used in PBD.

Fig. 9.1 Global minimum versus local minimum

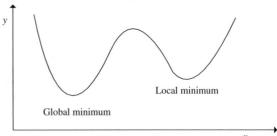

9.2 Genetic Algorithm

The genetic algorithm (GA) is a powerful evolutionary algorithm, based on the process of natural selection [1]. It uses techniques which perform heuristic searches that mimic the processes of natural evolution, such as reproduction, inheritance, crossover, mutation, and selection.

9.2.1 Flowchart

This heuristic process is routinely used to generate useful solutions to optimization problems. The individuals of GAs are encoded in the form of strings of chromosomes. Each chromosome is associated with a fitness function that represents the degree of fitness of the chromosome. A collection of individuals with such strings of chromosomes is called a population.

The flowchart of a GA is illustrated in Fig. 9.2:

- First, a random population is initially created to represent different candidates in the search space. Every individual is a complete solution to the jigsaw puzzle.
- Next, biologically inspired operators (crossover and mutation) are applied to those individuals.
- Third, a few best-fit individuals are selected with higher probabilities, to produce more offspring than other individuals. This selection gradually updates and improves the population in terms of their fitness values.
- The process iterates until the termination criteria are reached.

GAs differ from classical optimization techniques, such as gradient-based algorithms, in the following respects [2]. (1) GAs make use of the encoding of the parameters not the parameters themselves. (2) GAs work on a population of points

Fig. 9.2 Flowchart of a GA

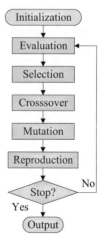

instead of a single point. (3) GAs use only the values of the objective function not their derivatives or other auxiliary knowledge. (4) GAs use probabilistic transition functions and not deterministic ones.

The Matlab command "ga" can find a minimum function. Table 9.3 shows its input and output arguments.

9.2.2   Evolutionary Algorithm

Three other important evolutionary algorithms are listed in Table 9.4. They are evolution strategy (ES), evolutionary programming (EP), and genetic programming (GP).

Table 9.3 The "ga" command

[x, fval, exitflag] = ga(fitnessfcn, nvars, A, b, Aeq, beq, LB, UB, nonlcon)
Input   fitnessfcn: fitness function   nvars: number of variables   A: matrix for linear inequality constraints   b: vector for linear inequality constraints   Aeq: matrix for linear equality constraints   beq: vector for linear equality constraints   LB: lower bound   UB: upper bound   nonlcon: non linear constraints
Output   x: best solution   fval: fitness function evaluated at x   exitflag: Reason why ga stopped iterating

Table 9.4 Important evolutionary algorithms

Method	Implementation
Evolution strategy	It evolves individuals by means of mutation and intermediate or discrete recombination. It uses self-adaptation to adjust the control parameters of the search
Evolutionary programming	It involves populations of solutions with primarily mutation and selection and arbitrary representations. It uses self-adaptation to adjust parameters, and can include other variation operations such as combining information from multiple parents
Genetic programming	It uses populations of computer programs. These complex computer programs are encoded in simpler linear chromosomes of fixed length, which are afterwards expressed as expression trees

9.3 Simulated Annealing

The simulated annealing (SA) algorithm is a probabilistic hill-climbing technique that is based on the annealing/cooling process of metals. This annealing process occurs after the heat source is removed from a molten metal and its temperature starts to decrease. As the temperature decreases, the energy of the metal molecules reduces, and the metal becomes more rigid. The procedure continues until the metal temperature has reached the surrounding ambient temperature, at which stage the energy has reached its lowest value and the metal is perfectly solid.

9.3.1 Algorithm

The SA procedure begins by generating an initial solution at random. At initial stages, a small random change is made in the current solution X_c. The new solution is called X_n. The perturbation depends on a temperate parameter T, and a scaling constant k:

$$pert(T) = k \times T \times r_3 \tag{9.1}$$

Here r_3 is a random value between 0 and 1 with uniform distribution. The temperature T decreases with each iteration of the algorithm, thus reducing the size of the perturbations as the search progresses. This mechanism produces a large perturbation in the initial stages of the search and ensures that the resulting parameters are fine-tuned toward the end of the optimization.

A move is made to the new solution X_n if it has smaller energy F or if the probability function has a higher value than a randomly generated number. Otherwise a new solution is generated, evaluated, and compared again. The probability p of accepting a new solution X_n which is called "Metropolis law" is given as follows:

$$p = \begin{cases} 1 & \text{if } F(X_n) < F(X_c) \\ \exp\left(\frac{F(X_c) - F(X_n)}{T}\right) & \text{otherwise} \end{cases} \tag{9.2}$$

In order to avoid getting trapped at local extrema, the reduction rate of T should be slow. In this study the following method, to reduce the temperature, has been used:

$$T_n = T_0 \times \beta^n \tag{9.3}$$

Here T_0 is the initial temperature; β is the reduction constant; and n is the number of iterations. In general, most worsening moves may be accepted at initial stages, but at the final stage only improving ones are likely to be allowed. This can

Table 9.5 The "simulannealbnd" command

[x, fval, exitflag] = simulannealbnd(fun, x0, lb, ub, options)
Input fun: function to be minimized x0: initial point lb: lower bound ub: upper bound options: optimization options
Output x: best solution fval: fitness function evaluated at x exitflag: Reason why ga stopped iterating

help the procedure jump out of a local minimum. Table 9.5 details the "simulannealbnd" command which can perform the SA algorithm in Matlab.

9.3.2 Restarted Simulated Annealing

However, sometimes it is better to move back to a former solution that was significantly better rather than always moving from the current state. This process is called "restarting" of SA.

To do this, we set the temperature to a former value and restart the annealing schedule. The decision to restart can be based on several criteria, including whether a fixed number of steps has passed or whether the current energy is too high compared with the best obtained so far, or simply the requirement for a random restart. The flowchart of restarted simulated annealing (RSA) is shown in Fig. 9.3.

Fig. 9.3 Diagram of RSA

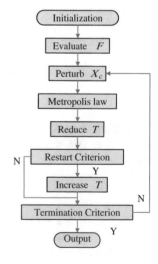

9.4 Tabu Search

The tabu search (TS) is a mathematical optimization method, belonging to the class of local search techniques. It enhances the performance of a local search method by using memory structures: once a potential solution has been determined, it is marked as "tabu" so that the algorithm does not visit that possibility repeatedly.

9.4.1 Description

The TS uses a local or neighborhood search procedure to iteratively move from a solution x to a solution x' in the neighborhood of x, until some stopping criterion has been satisfied. To explore regions of the search space that would be left unexplored by the local search procedure, TS modifies the neighborhood structure of each solution as the search progresses.

The solutions admitted to $N^*(x)$, the new neighborhood, are determined through the use of memory structures. The search then progresses by iteratively moving from a solution x to a solution x' in $N^*(x)$. The most important type of memory structure used to determine the solutions admitted to $N^*(x)$ is called the "tabu list (TL)." The TL is a short-term memory containing the solutions that have been visited in the recent past, less than n iterations ago in the program, where n is the number of previous solutions to be stored and n is also called the tabu tenure.

9.4.2 Memory Type

The memory structure in the TS are segmented into three categories:

1. short-term memory;
2. intermediate memory; and
3. long-term memory.

Short-term memory only stores recently considered solutions, which are not revisited until the expiration deactivates. The intermediate memory stores intensification rules, which aim to search toward promising areas. Long-term memory stores diversification rules, which drive the search into new regions.

9.5   Artificial Immune System

All living organisms have an immune system, the complexity of which depends on the species. When an attack by pathogens occurs, immune cells try to recognize and eliminate the them.

9.5.1   Receptor–Ligand Binding

How do immune cells recognize a specific pathogen from thousands of different shapes? Antibodies have unique binding requirements. When ligands of antigens and receptors of antibodies have complementary shapes (Fig. 9.4), they can bind together. The strength of the binding is called "*affinity*" [3].

The receptor–ligand binding [4] is highly specific, which enables the antibody to recognize disease-causing pathogens or non-self substances. The binding ensures recognition and then the immune system commences its response.

9.5.2   Human Immune System

When a foreign antigen is introduced into the host's body, it is first processed by lymphocytic cells of the non-specific defense system. This sets off a sequential series of events that eventually acts on a small population of randomly produced B-cells and T-cells, happening to have on their surface, antibodies that bind to the foreign antigen.

These trigger a rapid proliferation of both B-cell and T-cell populations, producing a large number of clones. These cell-clones differentiate into plasma cells

Fig. 9.4 Receptor–ligand binding

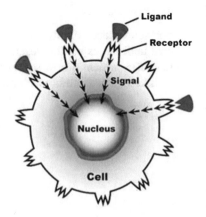

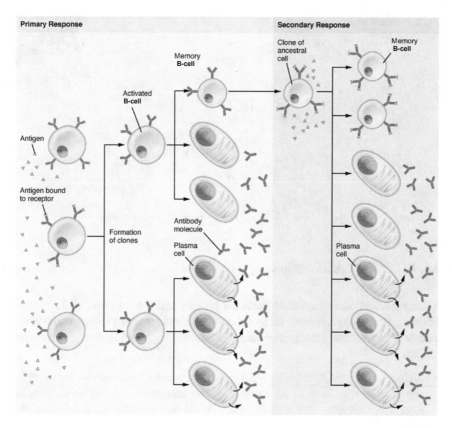

Fig. 9.5 The clonal selection principle

that are antibody-producing factories, spewing out prodigious quantities of one specific antibody, which binds to the specific antigen-epitope that stimulated it.

The specific antibody floods through the host. Wherever it binds to its epitope, it marks it for attacking and destroying by appropriate cells and associated components of the immune system.

Figure 9.5 shows that the specific antibodies are selected, and then differentiated into long-lived memory cells. These memory cells remain in the system although the foreign antigen is removed.

9.5.3 Remembering Response

Once the original antigen again appears in the host, these memory cells respond rapidly and produce even higher levels of antibodies. It is this "remembering response" that means hosts remain immune to many diseases for a long time, as shown in Fig. 9.6.

Fig. 9.6 Remembering
response

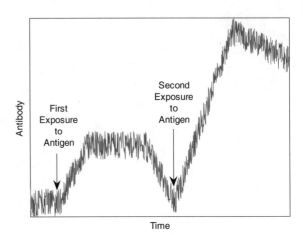

9.5.4 Affinity Maturation

Affinity maturation is the whole mutation process and the selection of the variant offspring that recognizes the antigen better than others. Those two fundamental mechanisms of affinity maturation are abbreviated as: hypermutation and receptor editing.

- *Mutations* take place in the variable regions of genes of antibodies. Occasionally one change may lead to an increase in the affinity of the antibody. Somatic hypermutation rate is inversely proportional to cell affinity: the higher the affinity a cell receptor has with an antigen, the lower the mutation rate, and vice versa. Under this strategy, the immune system keeps in hand the high-affinity offspring cells and also ensures large mutations for low-affinity ones in order to attain better affinity of cells.
- However, a large proportion of mutating antibodies may become non-functional or even anti-self cells due to the random mutation processes. Fortunately, there is a known process, *receptor editing*, which helps to remove these harmful cells.

9.5.5 Algorithms

Inspired by the human immune system, we can obtain a rough pipeline diagram of the artificial immune system (AIS) (Fig. 9.7).

Four main techniques were derived from the AIS concept. They are the clonal selection algorithm (CSA), the negative selection algorithm (NSA) [5], the immune network algorithm (INA) [6], and the dendritic cell algorithm (DCA) [7].

Fig. 9.7 Pipeline diagram for
an AIS

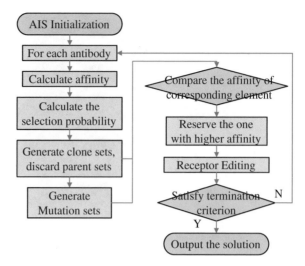

9.6   Particle Swarm Optimization

Particle swarm optimization (PSO) is a famous swarm intelligence (SI) method. It
mimics the behavior and movement of birds flocking or fish schooling, as shown in
Figs. 9.8 and 9.9, respectively.

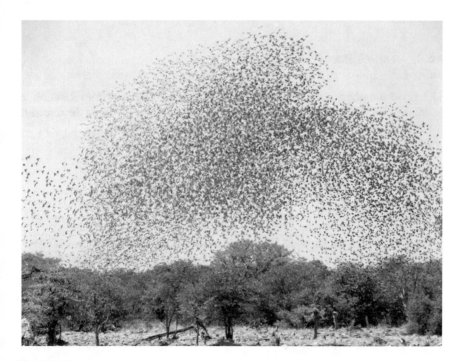

Fig. 9.8 Birds flocking

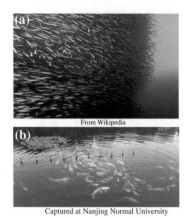

Fig. 9.9 Examples of fish schooling

9.6.1 Swarm Intelligence Principal

Millonas [8] at the Santa Fe Institute proposed five principles that SI must satisfy. They are the: proximity principle, quality principle, diverse response principle, stability principle, and adaptability principle [9]. Their meanings are listed in Table 9.6.

9.6.2 Algorithm

PSO performs searching via a swarm of particles that updates from iteration to iteration [10, 11]. To seek the optimal solution, each particle moves in the direction to its previously best (*pbest*) position and the global best (*gbest*) position in the swarm:

Table 9.6 Principles of SI

Principle	Definition
Proximity	The swarm should be able to do simple space and time computations
Quality	The swarm should be able to respond to quality factors in the environment
Diverse response	The swarm should not commit its activities along excessively narrow channels
Stability	The swarm should not change its mode of behavior every time the environment changes
Adaptability	The swarm should be able to change its behavior mode when it is worth the computational price to do so

$$pbest(i,t) = \underset{k=1,\ldots,t}{\arg \min}[f(P_i(k))], \quad i \in \{1,2,\ldots,N_P\} \tag{9.4}$$

$$gbest(t) = \underset{\substack{i=1,\ldots,N_P \\ k=1,\ldots,t}}{\arg \min}[f(P_i(k))] \tag{9.5}$$

where i denotes the particle index; N_P the total number of particles; t the current iteration number; f the fitness function; and P the position. The velocity V and position P of particles are updated by the following equations:

$$V_i(t+1) = \omega V_i(t) + c_1 r_1(pbest(i,t) - P_i(t)) + c_2 r_2(gbest(t) - P_i(t)) \tag{9.6}$$

$$P_i(t+1) = P_i(t) + V_i(t+1) \tag{9.7}$$

where V denotes the velocity; ω is the inertia weight used to balance global exploration and local exploitation; r_1 and r_2 are uniformly distributed random variables within range [0, 1]; and c_1 and c_2 are positive constant parameters called "acceleration coefficients" [12]. The meaning of Eq. (9.6) is offered in Table 9.7.

It is common to set an upper bound for the velocity parameter. "Velocity clamping" is used as a way to limit particles flying out of the search space. Another method is the "constriction coefficient" strategy, proposed by Clerc and Kennedy [13], as an outcome of a theoretical analysis of swarm dynamics, in which velocities are constricted too.

The pseudocode of PSO is listed in Table 9.8. Some important modifications of PSO are as follows: quantum-behaved PSO, bare-bones PSO, chaotic PSO, fuzzy PSO, PSO with a time-varying acceleration coefficient, opposition-based PSO, topology based PSO, etc.

Table 9.7 Meaning of the terms in Eq. (9.6)

Part	Term	Meaning
First	$\omega V_i(t)$	Known as the "inertia" component; it represents the previous velocity, which provides the necessary momentum for particles to roam across the search space
Middle	$c_1 r_1(pbest(i,t) - P_i(t))$	Known as the "cognitive" component; it represents the individual particle thinking about each of the other particles. It encourages the particles to move toward their own best positions found so far
Last	$c_2 r_2(gbest(t) - P_i(t))$	Known as the "cooperation" component; it represents the collaborative effect of the particles to find a global optimal solution

Table 9.8 Pseudocode of PSO

Step 1 Initialization

Step 1 Initialization

For each particle $i = 1, ..., N_P$, do

    a. Initialize the particle's position with a uniformly distribution as $P_i(0) \sim U(LB, UB)$, where LB and UB represent the lower and upper bounds of the search space

    b. Initialize *pbest* to its initial position: $pbest(i, 0) = P_i(0)$.

    c. Initialize *gbest* to the minimal value of the swarm: $gbest(0) = \arg\min f[P_i(0)]$.

    d. Initialize velocity: $V_i \sim U(-|UB - LB|, |UB - LB|)$.

Step 2 Repeat until a termination criteria is met

For each particle $i = 1, ..., N_P$, do

    a. Pick random numbers: $r_1, r_2 \sim U(0, 1)$.

    b. Update particle's velocity. See formula (9.6).

    c. Update particle's position. See formula (9.7).

    d. If $f[P_i(t)] < f[pbest(i, t)]$, do

        i. Update the best known position of particle i: $pbest(i, t) = P_i(t)$.

        ii. If $f[P_i(t)] < f[gbest(t)]$, update the swarm's best known position: $gbest(t) = P_i(t)$.

    e. $t \leftarrow (t + 1)$;

Step 3 Output *gbest(t)* that holds the best found solution.

9.6.3 Parallel Implementation

Parallel computing is a computational form, in which computations are carried out simultaneously.

- PSO can be implemented on multicore (multiprocessor) conditions.
- PSO can be implemented on a graphics processing unit (GPU) [14], which is a specialized electronic circuit designed to rapidly manipulate and alter memory to accelerate the creation of images in a frame buffer intended for output to a display.
- PSO can be implemented on cloud computing [15], which is a computing from in which large groups of remote servers are networked to allow centralized data storage and online access to computer services or resources.

9.7 Artificial Bee Colony

In nature, each bee only performs one single task, whereas, through a variety of information communication methods between bees, such as waggle dancing and release of special odors [16], the entire bee colony can easily find food resources

Fig. 9.10 An individual bee

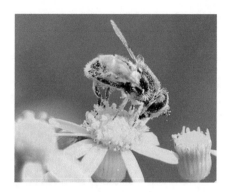

Fig. 9.11 A bee colony

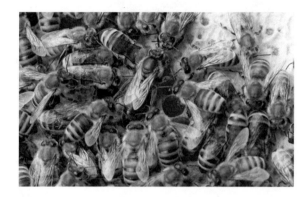

which produce relative high amounts of nectar [17], hence the colony realizes a self-organizing behavior (Figs. 9.10 and 9.11).

9.7.1   Components of a Honey Bee Colony

In order to introduce the self-organization model of forage selection that leads to the emergence of collective intelligence within a honey bee colony [18], we should define four essential components (Table 9.9).

9.7.2   Pseudocode

The diagram of the ABC algorithm is shown in Fig. 9.12. The detailed main steps of the algorithm are given below.

Table 9.9 Four components in an artificial bee colony (ABC) algorithm

Component	Purpose
Food resource	The value of a food source depends on different parameters, such as its proximity to the nest, its richness in terms of concentration of energy, and the ease by which this energy can be extracted. For simplicity, the profitability of a food source can be represented with a single quantity
Scout	If a bee starts searching spontaneously without any knowledge, it is known as a scout bee. The percentage of scout bees varies from 5 to 30% according to information from different nests. The mean number of scouts, averaged over different conditions, is about 10% of the colony, in nature
Onlooker	Onlookers wait in the nest and find a food source through the information shared by employed foragers. If onlookers attend a waggle dance done by some other bee, the bees become recruits and start searching by using the knowledge gained from the waggle dance
Employed forager	Employed foragers are associated with a particular food source, which they are currently exploiting or are "employed" at. They carry with them information about this particular source, its distance and direction from the nest, and the profitability of the source. They share this information with a certain probability. After the employed foraging bee loads a portion of nectar from the food source, it returns to the hive and unloads the nectar to the food area in the hive

Fig. 9.12 Diagram of the ABC algorithm

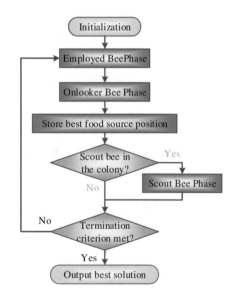

Step 1 Initialize the population of solutions x_{ij} (here i denotes the i-th solution and j denotes the j-th epoch, $i = 1, \ldots,$ SN, here SN denotes the number of solutions) with $j = 0$:

$$x_{i0} = \text{LB} + \text{rand}() \times (\text{UB} - \text{LB}) \quad (i = 1, \ldots, \text{SN}) \tag{9.8}$$

here LB and UB represent the lower and upper bounds, which can be infinity if not specified. Then, evaluate the population via the specified optimization function.

Step 2 Repeat, and let $j = j + 1$.

Step 3 Produce new solutions (food source positions) v_{ij} in the neighborhood of x_{ij} for the employed bees using the formula:

$$v_{ij} = x_{ij} + \Phi_{ij}(x_{ij} - x_{kj}) \tag{9.9}$$

where x_{kj} is a randomly chosen solution in the neighborhood of x_{ij} to produce a mutant of solution x_{ij} and Φ is a random number in the range $[-1, 1]$. Evaluate the new solutions.

Step 4 Apply the greedy selection process between the corresponding x_{ij} and v_{ij}.

Step 5 Calculate the probability values P_{ij} for the solutions x_{ij} by means of their fitness values using the equation:

$$P_{ij} = \frac{f_{ij}}{\sum_{i=1}^{\text{SN}} f_{ij}} \tag{9.10}$$

where f denotes the fitness value.

Step 6 Normalize P_{ij} values into $[0, 1]$.

Step 7 Produce the new solutions (new positions) v_{ij} for the onlookers from the solutions x_{ij} using the same equation as in Step 3, selected depending on P_{ij}, and evaluate them.

Step 8 Apply the greedy selection process for the onlookers between x_{ij} and v_{ij}.

Step 9 Determine the abandoned solution (source), if it exists, and replace it with a new randomly produced solution x_{ij} for the scout using the equation:

$$x_{ij} = \min_i(x_{ij}) + \varphi_{ij} * \left(\max_i(x_{ij}) - \min_i(x_{ij}) \right) \tag{9.11}$$

where φ_{ij} is a random number in $[0, 1]$.

Step 10 Memorize the best food source position (solution) achieved so far.

Step 11 Go to Step 2 until termination criteria is met.

9.8   Firefly Algorithm

The firefly algorithm (FA) is an algorithm inspired by nature, based on the flashing behavior of a firefly swarm (Figs. 9.13 and 9.14).

9.8.1   Rule

The primary purpose of the flash made by fireflies is to signal to, and attract, other fireflies. The FA consists of three rules [19]:

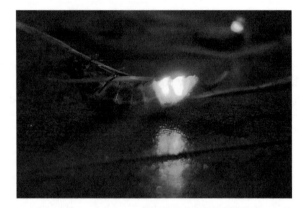

Fig. 9.13 A individual firefly

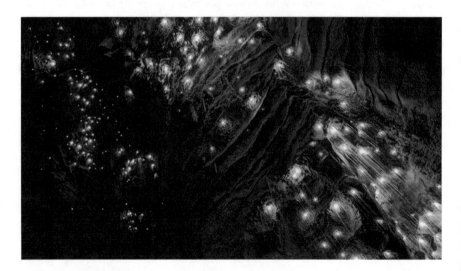

Fig. 9.14 A firefly swarm

- All fireflies are unisex so that one firefly will be attracted to other fireflies regardless of their sex.
- An important and interesting behavior of fireflies is to glow brighter mainly to attract prey and to share food with others.
- Attractiveness is proportional to their brightness; thus, each agent first moves toward a neighbor that glows brighter.

9.8.2   Algorithm

In the FA, the fireflies are randomly distributed in the search space. The fireflies carry a luminescence quality, called luciferin, which emits light proportional to its quality [20]. Each firefly is attracted to the brighter glow of other approximated fireflies. The attractiveness decreases as their distance increases. If there is no brighter glow within the scope of a particular firefly, it will move randomly in the search space [21].

The brightness is related to objective values, so for an optimization problem, a firefly with higher intensity will attract another firefly with higher probability, and vice versa. Assume that there exists a swarm of n fireflies and x_i represents a solution for a firefly i, whereas $f(x_i)$ denotes its corresponding energy value. Here the brightness I of a firefly is equivalent to the simplified energy value:

$$I_i = f(x_i), \quad 1 \leq i \leq n \tag{9.12}$$

The attractiveness β of the firefly is proportional to the light intensity received by adjacent fireflies [22]. Suppose β_0 is the attractiveness with distance $r = 0$, so for two fireflies i and j at locations x_i and x_j, their attractiveness is calculated as:

$$\beta_r(i,j) = \beta_0 \exp\left\{-\gamma r(i,j)^2\right\} \tag{9.13}$$

$$r(i,j) = \left\|x_i - x_j\right\| \tag{9.14}$$

where $r(i, j)$ denotes the distance between fireflies i and j; and γ denotes the light absorption coefficient. Suppose firefly j is brighter than firefly i, then firefly i will move to a new location as:

$$x_i(t+1) = x_i(t) + \beta_0 \exp\left\{-\gamma r^2\right\}(x_j - x_i) \tag{9.15}$$

The pseudocode of the FA is summarized in Table 9.10.

Table 9.10 Pseudocode of the FA

Step 1 Initialization.
Step 1.1 Create the initial population of n fireflies $(x_1, x_2, \ldots,$ and $x_n)$ within d-dimensional search space.
Step 1.2 Formulate light intensity of each firefly so as to be associated with the energy value $f(x)$.
Step 1.3 Define the parameters β_0 and γ.
Step 2 Perform.
while (termination criteria are not met)
for $i = 1$ to n
for $j = 1$ to n
if $(I_j < I_i)$
Move firefly j towards firefly i via Eq. (9.15).
end if
Update attractiveness table.
Evaluate new solutions and update light intensity.
end for j
end for i
Rank the fireflies and find the best.
end for while
Step 3 Post-processing and output.

9.9   Ant Colony Optimization

Ant colony optimization (ACO) is an algorithm developed recently to simulate the behavior of real ants (Fig. 9.15) to rapidly establish the shortest route from a food source to their nest and vice versa [23].

Ants begin randomly searching for food in the area surrounding their nest. When an individual ant encounters food along its path, it deposits a small quantity of pheromone at that location. Other ants in the neighborhood detect this marked pheromone trail. As more ants follow the pheromone-rich trail, the probability of

Fig. 9.15 An individual ant

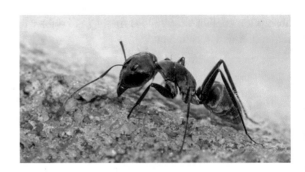

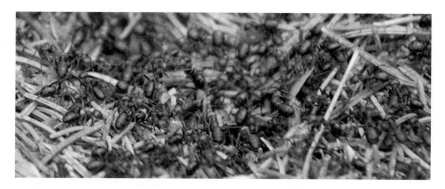

Fig. 9.16 An ant colony

the trial being followed by other ants is further enhanced by increased pheromone deposition. Figure 9.16 presents part of an ant colony seeking food.

9.9.1   Algorithm

This auto catalytic process reinforced by a positive feedback mechanism helps the ants to establish a shortest route [24]. The pipeline of the algorithm is stated as follows.

Suppose we have an undirected graph $G = (O, A)$, where O is the set of nodes and A is the set of arcs connecting the nodes. The density of the nodes determines both the precision of a solution and the memory and computation time demands of the algorithm. All arcs O are initialized with a small amount of pheromone τ_0. The target is to find the shortest path from the source node O_1 to the destination node O_2.

Next, N ants are sequentially launched from O_1, where N is the number of ants in the colony. Each ant walks pseudo-randomly from node to node via connecting arcs as far as the O_2, or to the point a dead end is reached. When deciding which node x to go to from a specific node y, the probability P_{xy} is assigned as follows:

$$P_{xy} = \frac{\tau_{xy}(k)^{\alpha}\eta_{xy}(k)^{\beta}}{\sum_{y \in \text{allowed}_y} \tau_{xy}(k)^{\alpha}\eta_{xy}(k)^{\beta}} \qquad (9.16)$$

Here the trail level $\tau_{xy}(k)$ is the amount of pheromone currently available at step k in the arc from node x to node y. It indicates how proficient the ant has been in the past to make the move from x to y. The attractiveness $\eta_{xy}(k)$ is the desirability of the move from x to y. Parameters α and β control the relative importance of the trail level and attractiveness, respectively. The trail levels of all arcs are updated according to moves that were part of "good" or "bad" solutions:

$$\tau_{xy}(k+1) = \begin{cases} (1-\rho)[\tau_{xy}(k)+Q], & (x,y) \in BestRoute \\ (1-\rho)\tau_{xy}(k), & (x,y) \notin BestRoute \end{cases} \qquad (9.17)$$

Here ρ denotes the pheromone evaporation coefficient and Q a pheromone constant. Pheromone evaporation also has the advantage of avoiding the convergence to a locally optimal solution. If there were no evaporation at all, the paths chosen by the first ants would tend to be excessively attractive to the following ones.

At any iteration, the best route is calculated from N routes. The pheromones of the best route are enforced while others evaporate. It should be noted that local updates exist in some models; however, the models with local updates cannot guarantee convergence.

9.9.2   Extension to a Continuous Problem

Note that a combinatory optimization problem can be solved directly by ACO, however, our mission is a continuous space optimization problem, so ACO cannot be directly used to solve our problem. A special coding strategy can be used to transform the continuous space into the routine search problem. Figure 9.17 gives a simple example, coding the value 4.85 as a routine.

Fig. 9.17 Coding strategy for ACO solving continuous optimization

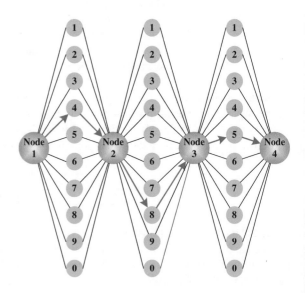

9.10 Biogeography-Based Optimization

Biogeography-based optimization (BBO) was inspired by biogeography, which describes speciation (i.e., the formation of new and distinct species in the course of evolution [25]) and migration of species between isolated habitats (such as the island location shown in Fig. 9.18) as well as the extinction of species.

9.10.1 Habitat

Habitats friendly to life are termed to have a high habitat suitability index (HSI), and vice versa. Features that correlate with the HSI include land area, rainfall, topographic diversity, temperature, vegetative diversity, etc. These features are called suitability index variables (SIV). Like other biology-inspired algorithms, the SIV and HSI are considered as search space and objective function, respectively [26].

9.10.2 Migration

Habitats with a high HSI have not only a high emigration rate [27], but also a low immigration rate, because they already support many species. Species that migrate to this kind of habitat will tend to die even if it has high HSI, because there is too much competition for resources from other species. On the other hand, habitats with a low HSI have both a high emigration rate and a low immigration rate; the reason is not because species want to immigrate, but because there are a lot of resources available for additional species [28].

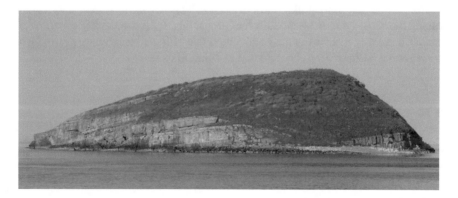

Fig. 9.18 An isolated island

Fig. 9.19 Model of
immigration λ and emigration
μ probabilities

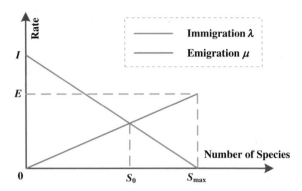

To illustrate, Fig. 9.19 shows the relationship between immigration and emigration probabilities, where λ and μ represent immigration and emigration probabilities, respectively. I and E represent the maximum immigration and emigration rates, respectively. S_{max} is the maximum number of species the habitat can support, and S_0 the equilibrium species count. Following common convention, we assume a linear relation between rates and number of species, and give the definition of immigration and emigration rates of habitats that contains S species as follows:

$$\lambda_S = I\left(1 - \frac{S}{S_{max}}\right) \tag{9.18}$$

$$\mu_S = \frac{ES}{S_{max}} \tag{9.19}$$

The emigration and immigration rates are used to share information between habitats. Consider the special case $E = I$, we have:

$$\lambda_S + \mu_S = E \tag{9.20}$$

Emigration and immigration rates of each habitat are used to share information among the ecosystem. With modification probability P_{mod}, we modify solutions H_i and H_j in the way that we use the immigration rate of H_i and emigration rate of H_j to decide some SIVs of H_j to be migrated to some SIVs of H_i.

9.10.3 Mutation and Elitism

Mutation is simulated in the SIV level. Very high and very low HSI solutions are equally improbable, nevertheless, medium HSI solutions are relatively probable. The above idea can be implemented as a mutation rate m, which is inversely proportional to the solution probability P_S:

Table 9.11 Pseudocode of BBO

Step 1 Initialize BBO parameters, which include a problem-dependent method of mapping problem solutions to SIVs and habitats, the modification probability P_{mod}, the maximum species count S_{max}, the maximum migration rates E and I, the maximum mutation rate m_{max}, and the elite number p.
Step 2 Initialize a random set of habitats.
Step 3 Compute HSI for each habitat.
Step 4 Computer S, λ, and μ for each habitat.
Step 5 Modify the whole ecosystem by migration based on P_{mod}, λ, and μ.
Step 6 Mutate the ecosystem based on mutate probabilities.
Step 7 Implement elitism.
Step 8 If termination criterion was met, output the best habitat, otherwise jump to Step 3.

$$m(H) = m_{max}\left(\frac{1 - \mathbf{P}_S}{\mathbf{P}_{max}}\right) \qquad (9.21)$$

where m_{max} is a user-defined parameter, representing the maximum mutation rate. $\mathbf{P}_{max}$ is the maximum value of $\mathbf{P}(\infty)$.

Elitism was also included in standard BBO, in order to retain the best solutions in the ecosystem. Hence, the mutation approach will not impair the high HSI habitats. Elitism is implemented by setting $\lambda = 0$ for the p best habitats, where p is a predefined elitism parameter. In closing, the pseudocode of BBO is listed in Table 9.11.

9.10.4 Pseudocode

As shown in Fig. 9.20, BBO is similar to the GA: each chromosome in the GA is considered an SIV in BBO. The individual in the GA is the habitat in BBO. Population corresponds to ecosystem. Fitness value is referred to as HSI. Table 9.11 presents the pseudocode of BBO.

Fig. 9.20 Relationship between the GA and BBO

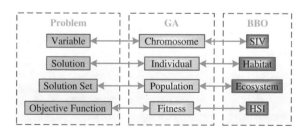

9.11 Jaya Algorithm

For the above meta-heuristic approaches, they usually obtain better performances than BP and its variants, however, they need to tune both common controlling parameters (CCPs) and algorithm-specific parameters (ASPs), which influence their performance and complicate their applications.

Recently, a novel approach, called Jaya (a Sanskrit word meaning victory) was proposed by Rao [29], which does not need to tune ASPs, but only needs to set their values (typically the population size and maximum iteration number). The authors compared Jaya with the latest approaches, and they found Jaya ranks first for "best" and "mean" solutions for all 24 constrained benchmark problems, and gives better performances over 30 unconstrained benchmark problems.

Figure 9.21 shows a flowchart for Jaya. Here suppose b and w represent the index of the best and worst candidate among the population, and suppose i, j, and k is the index of iteration, variable, and candidate. Then $V(i, j, k)$ means the j-th variable of the k-th candidate in the i-th iteration. The modification formula of each candidate can be written as:

$$V(i+1,j,k) = V(i,j,k)$$
$$+ r(i,j,1)(V(i,j,b) - |V(i,j,k)|) - r(i,j,2)(V(i,j,w) - |V(i,j,k)|)$$
$$(9.22)$$

Fig. 9.21 Flowchart of the Jaya algorithm

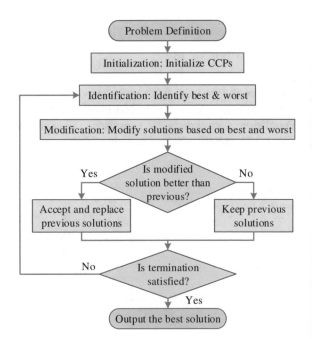

where $V(i, j, b)$ and $V(i, j, w)$ represent the best and worst value of the j-th variable in the i-th iteration. The $r(i, j, 1)$ and $r(i, j, 2)$ are two positive numbers in the range of [0, 1], generated at random. The second term "$r(i, j, 1)(V(i, j, b) - |V(i, j, k)|$" indicates the candidate should move closer to the best one, while the third term "$-r(i, j, 2)(V(i, j, w) - |V(i, j, k)|$" indicates that the candidate should move further away from the worst one (note the minus symbol before r). The $V(i + 1, j, k)$ is accepted if the modified candidate is better in terms of function values, otherwise the previous $V(i, j, k)$ is maintained.

9.12 Early Stopping

Readers should notice that the optimization algorithms for training classifiers is different from traditional optimization algorithms, namely, the training is not a "*pure*" optimization problem.

The training is to minimize the loss on the training set. Hence, the error is named empirical risk minimization (ERM). What we really seek is to minimize the error on new data, and in practice we use validation error instead.

Practically, the early stopping technique is used. Here Fig. 9.22 shows that at epoch 6, the validation error reaches a minimum. Then from the 6th to the 11th epoch, we observe validation increasing although the training error decreases, which indicates that an overfitting has occurred. Hence, we should select the weights corresponding to the 6th epoch. In addition, it suggests that is not necessary to set the maximum epoch number for classifier training.

Fig. 9.22 Example of early stopping

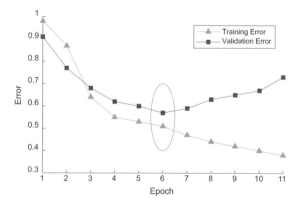

9.13 Conclusion

In this chapter, the canonical backpropagation gradient descent algorithm, and its variants, were introduced. Ten biologically inspired algorithms: the genetic algorithm, simulated annealing, the tabu search, the artificial immune system, particle swarm optimization, the artificial bee colony, the firefly algorithm, ant colony optimization, biogeography-based optimization, and the Jaya algorithm were presented and compared.

There are other interesting global optimization algorithms, for instance, the cat swarm optimization [30], etc. The hybridization of these algorithms is expected to give better performance than the original algorithms [31]. Swarm intelligence is an important research direction that is attracting the attention of more and more scholars. Readers are encouraged to download their codes on the internet and test their performance. Note that the training of classifier is not a pure optimization problem; hence, early stopping is often used as a stopping criterion.

References

1. Tan JZ, Kerr WL (2017) Determination of glass transitions in boiled candies by capacitance based thermal analysis (CTA) and genetic algorithm (GA). J Food Eng 193:68–75. https://doi.org/10.1016/j.jfoodeng.2016.08.010
2. Nguyen P, Kim JM (2016) Adaptive ECG denoising using genetic algorithm-based thresholding and ensemble empirical mode decomposition. Inf Sci 373:499–511. https://doi.org/10.1016/j.ins.2016.09.033
3. Jun Y, Wei G (2010) Find multi-objective paths in stochastic networks via chaotic immune PSO. Expert Syst Appl 37(3):1911–1919
4. Laffitte A, Neiers F, Brockhoff A, Meyerhof W, Briand L (2016) Interaction of the human T1R2 taste receptor ligand-binding domain with sweeteners and sweet-tasting proteins. Chem Senses 41(9):E124–E124
5. Guevara CB, Santos M, Lopez V (2016) Negative selection and Knuth Morris Pratt Algorithm for anomaly detection. IEEE Latin Am Trans 14(3):1473–1479
6. Abo-Zahhad M, Sabor N, Sasaki S, Ahmed SM (2016) A centralized immune-Voronoi deployment algorithm for coverage maximization and energy conservation in mobile wireless sensor networks. Inf Fusion 30:36–51. https://doi.org/10.1016/j.inffus.2015.11.005
7. Chelly Z, Elouedi Z (2016) A survey of the dendritic cell algorithm. Knowl Inf Syst 48 (3):505–535. https://doi.org/10.1007/s10115-015-0891-y
8. Millonas M (1994) Swarms, phase transitions and collective intelligence. In: Langton C (ed) Artificial life III. Addison-Wesley, Reading, MA, pp 417–445
9. Ji G (2015) A comprehensive survey on particle swarm optimization algorithm and its applications. Math Probl Eng, Article ID: 931256
10. Lahmiri S (2017) Glioma detection based on multi-fractal features of segmented brain MRI by particle swarm optimization techniques. Biomed Signal Process Control 31:148–155. https://doi.org/10.1016/j.bspc.2016.07.008
11. Yang JF, Sun P (2016) Magnetic resonance brain classification by a novel binary particle swarm optimization with mutation and time-varying acceleration coefficients. Biomed Eng-Biomed Tech 61(4):431–441. https://doi.org/10.1515/bmt-2015-0152

12. Tawhid MA, Ali AF (2016) Simplex particle swarm optimization with arithmetical crossover for solving global optimization problems. Opsearch 53(4):705–740. https://doi.org/10.1007/s12597-016-0256-7
13. Clerc M, Kennedy J (2002) The particle swarm-explosion, stability, and convergence in a multidimensional complex space. IEEE Trans Evol Comput 6(1):58–73. https://doi.org/10.1109/4235.985692
14. Narjess D, Sadok B (2016) A new hybrid GPU-PSO approach for solving Max-CSPs. In: Proceedings of the 2016 genetic and evolutionary computation conference, Denver, CO. ACM, pp 119–120. https://doi.org/10.1145/2908961.2908973
15. Alkhashai HM, Omara FA (2016) BF-PSO-TS: hybrid heuristic algorithms for optimizing task schedulingon cloud computing environment. Int J Adv Comput Sci Appl 7(6):207–212
16. Scaria A, George K, Sebastian J (2016) An artificial bee colony approach for multi-objective job shop scheduling. Proc Technol 25:1030–1037. https://doi.org/10.1016/j.protcy.2016.08.203
17. Wu L (2011) Optimal multi-level thresholding based on maximum Tsallis entropy via an artificial bee colony approach. Entropy 13(4):841–859
18. Lozano M, Garcia-Martinez C, Rodriguez FJ, Trujillo HM (2017) Optimizing network attacks by artificial bee colony. Inf Sci 377:30–50. https://doi.org/10.1016/j.ins.2016.10.014
19. Wu L (2013) Solving two-dimensional HP model by firefly algorithm and simplified energy function. Math Probl Eng, Article ID: 398141. https://doi.org/10.1155/2013/398141
20. Kaushik A, Tayal DK, Yadav K, Kaur A (2016) Integrating firefly algorithm in artificial neural network models for accurate software cost predictions. J Softw-Evol Process 28 (8):665–688. https://doi.org/10.1002/smr.1792
21. Brasileiro I, Santos I, Soares A, Rabelo R, Mazullo F (2015) Ant colony optimization applied to the problem of choosing the best combination among M combinations of shortest paths in transparent optical networks. In: IEEE congress on evolutionary computation (CEC), Sendai, Japan. IEEE, pp 259–266
22. Horng M-H (2012) Vector quantization using the firefly algorithm for image compression. Expert Syst Appl 39(1):1078–1091. https://doi.org/10.1016/j.eswa.2011.07.108
23. Taghizadeh-Mehrjardi R, Toomanian N, Khavaninzadeh AR, Jafari A, Triantafilis J (2016) Predicting and mapping of soil particle-size fractions with adaptive neuro-fuzzy inference and ant colony optimization in central Iran. Eur J Soil Sci 67(6):707–725. https://doi.org/10.1111/ejss.12382
24. Saraswathi K, Tamilarasi A (2016) Ant colony optimization based feature selection for opinion mining classification. J Med Imaging Health Inform 6(7):1594–1599. https://doi.org/10.1166/jmihi.2016.1856
25. Goudos SK (2016) A novel generalized oppositional biogeography-based optimization algorithm: application to peak to average power ratio reduction in OFDM systems. Open Math 14:705–722. https://doi.org/10.1515/math-2016-0066
26. Wei L (2015) Fruit classification by wavelet-entropy and feedforward neural network trained by fitness-scaled chaotic ABC and biogeography-based optimization. Entropy 17(8):5711–5728. https://doi.org/10.3390/e17085711
27. Crawford B, Soto R, Riquelme L, Olguin E (2016) Biogeography-based optimization algorithm for solving the set covering problem. In: Silhavy R, Senkerik R, Oplatkova ZK, Silhavy P, Prokopova Z (eds) 5th Computer science on-line conference (CSOC), prague advances in intelligent systems and computing. Springer, Berlin, pp 273–283. https://doi.org/10.1007/978-3-319-33625-1_25
28. Wu J (2016) Fruit classification by biogeography-based optimization and feedforward neural network. Expert Syst 33(3):239–253. https://doi.org/10.1111/exsy.12146
29. Rao RV (2016) Jaya: a simple and new optimization algorithm for solving constrained and unconstrained optimization problems. Int J Ind Eng Comput 7:19–34. https://doi.org/10.5267/j.ijiec.2015.8.004

30. Chu SC, Tsai PW, Pan JS (2006) Cat swarm optimization. In: Yang Q, Webb G (eds) 9th Pacific Rim international conference on artificial intelligence (PRICAI), Guilin, P.R. China. Lecture notes in artificial intelligence. Springer, Berlin, pp 854–858
31. Feng C (2015) Feed-forward neural network optimized by hybridization of PSO and ABC for abnormal brain detection. Int J Imaging Syst Technol 25(2):153–164. https://doi.org/10.1002/ima.22132

Chapter 10
Comparison of Artificial Intelligence–Based Pathological Brain Detection Systems

In this chapter, three data sets for single-slice pathological brain detection (PBD), along with their download URLs, are given. All the data sets can be downloaded from *The Whole Brain Atlas* from the Harvard Medical School. The inclusion criteria of three commonly used data sets are introduced. The limitation of using didactic images is explained. In the field of pattern recognition, a training set is necessary, where data are labelled using known categories. The validation set is important to optimize hyper-parameters. The performance over the test set is recorded for out-of-sample estimation. Nevertheless, data sizes are usually too small in PBD problems. Hence, cross-validation techniques are commonly used instead of holdout validation. Leave-p-out, leave-one-out, k-fold and its stratified version, and Monte Carlo cross validation are discussed and compared. The settings for k-fold stratified cross validation for the three data sets are given. For the first data set, k is assigned with a value of 6. For the other two data sets, k is assigned with a value of 5. A comparison is made of the 49 state-of-the-art methods in terms of employed features and classification accuracies. Their feature extraction methods, feature reduction methods, and classification methods are analyzed. Finally, the shortcomings of these latest PBD systems are discussed. Several feasible future directions are provided.

10.1 Three Single-Slice Data Sets

Single-slice PBD systems aim to make medical decisions based on one brain image. The image should contain lesions, otherwise the single-slice PBD system would have nothing to identify. Thus, the problem is how to detect the optimal slice containing the lesion.

Commonly used single-slice data sets can be downloaded from the homepage of *The Whole Brain Atlas* from the Harvard Medical School. Three inclusion criteria are listed:

© Springer Nature Singapore Pte Ltd. 2018

S.-H. Wang et al., *Pathological Brain Detection*, Brain Informatics and Health, https://doi.org/10.1007/978-981-10-4026-9_10

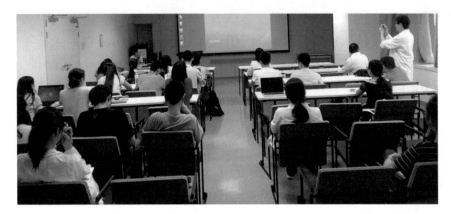

Fig. 10.1 A medicine lecture (didactic images usually have strong pathological features, which may not be observed easily in more realistic scenarios)

1. No more than five slices are selected from each subject (pathological or healthy).
2. The slices selected from patients should include lesions, confirmed by three radiologists with over ten years of experience.
3. The slices from healthy subjects are selected at random from the same range of patient slices.

   Three benchmark data sets (DI, DII, and DIII) are generated based on the collection of images mentioned above. The former two data sets (DI and DII) contain seven types of disease. DI consists of 66 images and DII consists of 160 images. The largest data set DIII contains 11 types of disease and 255 images.

   Note that the images on the Harvard Medical School website are mainly for didactic use. As such it only collects images from those patients with prominent abnormal features from otherwise healthy brains (Fig. 10.1). Hence, the performance across the data sets only reflects the algorithm's performance in ideal conditions, and it cannot reflect the algorithm's performance in real-world scenarios where the scanned images may be of poor quality.

10.2 Cross Validation

Unlike the millions of face images available to the field of face detection and classification, PBD systems contain far fewer images, usually dozens to hundreds of brain images. Therefore, it is not practical to divide the whole data set into training and test images. The cross validation technique is often used.

10.2.1 Leave-p-Out Cross Validation

The leave-p-out cross validation (LPOCV) uses p samples as the validation set, with the others being used as the training set. This is repeated to divide the original data set into two parts.

As is known, if the original data set contains n samples, then the LPOCV needs to learn and validate many times:

$$C_p^n = \frac{n!}{(n-p)!p!} \tag{10.1}$$

Here C represents the binomial coefficient.

Even for a small data set, for example, $n = 80$ and $p = 30$, we have:

$$C_{30}^{80} \approx 8.87 \times 10^{21} \tag{10.2}$$

10.2.2 Leave-One-Out Cross Validation

The leave-one-out cross validation (LOOCV) [2] is a particular case of LPOCV with $p = 1$. The LOOCV is similar to the jackknife technique. The difference is that the former computes a statistic on the left-out sample, while the latter computes a statistic from the kept samples only. The LOOCV does not take too much time, since:

$$C_1^n = n \tag{10.3}$$

10.2.3 k-Fold Cross Validation

The k-fold cross validation (kFCV) randomly partitions the whole data set into k folds. In each trial ($k-1$) is used as training, and the remaining folds as tests. This procedure repeats k times. In all, the k results over the test sets are combined to generate a single estimation. In some conditions, one fold is used for a test, one fold for validation, and the other ($k-2$) folds used for training.

Ten-fold cross validation is the most commonly used in PBD. Figure 10.2 shows ten-fold cross validation.

Stratification was often used in cross validation. By using stratification, the folds contain roughly the same proportions of class distribution. Suppose we have a 4-class 80-image dataset, and each class has exactly 20 images. The ordinary 10-fold cross validation randomly divide this dataset to 10 folds, but the stratified 10-fold cross validation will try to make each fold contains 2 images of each class.

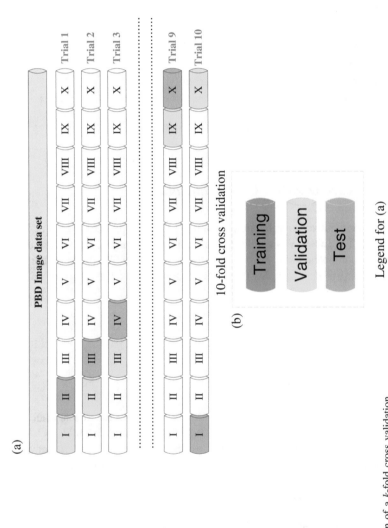

Fig. 10.2 Diagram of a *k*-fold cross validation

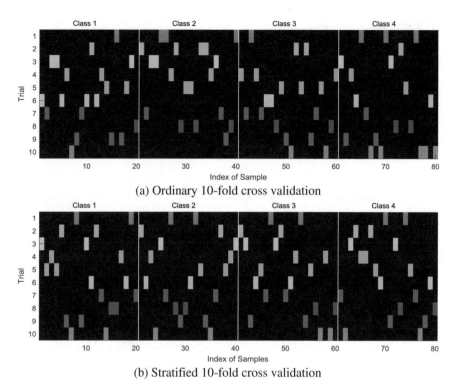

(a) Ordinary 10-fold cross validation

(b) Stratified 10-fold cross validation

Fig. 10.3 Comparison between ordinary and stratified cross validation

Figure 10.3a lists the ordinary 10-fold cross validation, where the first fold contains one C_1 sample, 3 C_2 samples, 1 C_3 sample, and 3 C_4 samples. Obviously, the class distribution in fold 1 is not even over all classes. Figure 10.3b shows the stratified one, showing each fold contains nearly the same class distribution.

10.2.4 Monte Carlo Cross Validation

The Monte Carlo cross validation (MCCV) randomly splits the data set [3]. In each case, the whole data set is split into either training or test. Compared to kFCV, the training/test portion of MCCV does not rely on the number of folds.

Nevertheless, some samples in MCCV may be selected in both training and test [4], and some samples may never be selected in either training or test. In all, the training and test sets in MCCV may overlap with each other.

10.2.5   Matlab Command

The Matlab command "crossvalind" is an important method used for cross validation. It has four types:

1. The *k*-fold type shown in Table 10.1.
2. The hold-out type shown in Table 10.2.
3. The leave-p-out type shown in Table 10.3.
4. The resubstitution type shown in Table 10.4.

Table 10.1 The "crossvalind" command for *k*-fold

Indices = crossvalind('Kfold', N, K)
Input N: number of observations K: k-fold
Output Indices[a]: contains approximately equal proportions of the integers 1 through K
[a]Define a partition of the N observations into K disjoint subsets

Table 10.2 The "crossvalind" command for hold-out

[Train, Test] = crossvalind('HoldOut', N, P)
Input N: number of observations P[a]: percentage of the test set
Output Train: training set Test: test set
[a]P should be between 0 and 1

Table 10.3 The "crossvalind" command for leave-*p*-out

[Train, Test] = crossvalind('LeaveMOut', N, M)
Input N: number of observations M: randomly select M observations to hold out for test set
Output Train: training set Test: test set

Table 10.4 The "crossvalind" command for resubstitution

[Train, Test] = crossvalind('Resubstitution', N, [P,Q])
Input N: number of observations P: randomly select P*N observation for test set Q: randomly select Q*N observation for training
Output Train: training set Test: test set

Table 10.5 SCV settings

Data set	k	Training		Validation		Total	
		H	P	H	P	H	P
DI	6	15	40	3	8	18	48
DII	5	16	112	4	28	20	140
DIII	5	28	176	7	44	35	220

k represents the number of folds, H healthy, P pathological

10.3   Statistical Analysis

The k-fold stratified cross validation (SCV) is commonly used. Compared to the standard cross validation, stratification rearranges the data so that each fold is fully representative of the whole data set. Usually, three benchmark data sets are divided in the way shown in Table 10.5.

To further reduce the randomness, the k-fold SCV can be run more than once. Traditionally, the k-fold SCV is run five times. In recent years, 10 repetitions were found to give more accurate results than 5 repititions.

10.4   Comparison of State-of-the-Art Methods

We compare 49 state-of-the-art single-slice PBD systems in this book. We presented their system structures in Table 10.6, and their classification performances in Table 10.7.

Table 10.6 Comparison of the system structures of state-of-the-art single-Slice PBD systems

Approach	Feature	Dimensionality reduction	Classifier	Optimization method
Patnaik et al. [1]	DWT		SOM	
	DWT		SVM	
	DWT		SVM + IPOL	
	DWT		SVM + RBF	
El-Dahshan et al. [2]	DWT	PCA	FNN	
	DWT	PCA	kNN	
Wu [3]	DWT	PCA	FNN	SCG
Wu [4]	DWT	PCA	SVM	
	DWT	PCA	SVM + RBF	
Saritha et al. [5]	WE	SWP	PNN	
Das et al. [6]	RT	PCA	LS-SVM	

(continued)

Table 10.6 (continued)

Approach	Feature	Dimensionality reduction	Classifier	Optimization method
Yang [7]	DWTE		GEPSVM	
	DWTE		GEPSVM + RBF	
Zhou et al. [8]	WE		NBC	
Feng [9]	SWT	PCA	FNN	IABAP
	SWT	PCA	FNN	ABC-SPSO
	SWT	PCA	FNN	HPA
Phillips et al. [10]	WE		FNN	HBP
Sun [11]	WE + HMI		GEPSVM	
	WE + HMI		GEPSVM + RBF	
Liu [12]	SWT	PCA	GEPSVM	
	SWT	PCA	GEPSVM + RBF	
Liu [13]	WPSE		SVM	
	WPTE		SVM	
	WPSE		FSVM	
	WPTE		FSVM	
Yang et al. [14]	FRFE	WTT	NBC	
	FRFE	WTT	SVM	
	FRFE	WTT	GEPSVM	
	FRFE	WTT	TSVM	
Nayak et al. [15]	DWT	PPCA	ADBRF	
	DWT	PPCA	ADBRF	
Atangana [16]	SWE		FNN	HBP
Zhou et al. [17]	SWT	PCA	SVM + HPOL	
	SWT	PCA	SVM + IPOL	
	SWT	PCA	SVM + RBF	
Yang [18]	DTCWT	VE	SVM	
	DTCWT	VE	GEPSVM	
	DTCWT	VE	TSVM	
Yang, Sun [19]	WE		PNN	BPSO-MT
Sun [20]	FRFE		MLP	ARCBBO
	FRFE		DP-MLP	ARCBBO
	FRFE		BDB-MLP	ARCBBO
	FRFE		KC-MLP	ARCBBO
Chen [21]	MBD		SLFN	GA
	MBD		SLFN	PSO
	MBD		SLFN	ABC
	MBD		SLFN	FA
	MBD		SLFN	PSO-TTC

For explanations of the abbreviations see page xvii in this book as well as corresponding publications

Table 10.7 Comparison of classification performances of state-of-the-art single-slice PBD systems

Approach	Repetition number	Feature number	DI	DII	DIII
Patnaik et al. [1]	OLD	4761	94.00	93.17	91.65
	OLD	4761	96.15	95.38	94.05
	OLD	4761	98.00	97.15	96.37
	OLD	4761	98.00	97.33	96.18
El-Dahshan et al. [2]	OLD	7	97.00	96.98	95.29
	OLD	7	98.00	97.54	96.79
Wu [3]	OLD	19	100.00	99.27	98.82
Wu [4]	OLD	19	96.01	95.00	94.29
	OLD	19	100.00	99.38	98.82
Saritha et al. [5]	OLD	3	100.00	99.88	98.90
Das et al. [6]	OLD	9	100.00	100.00	99.39
Yang [7]	NEW	16	100.00	100.00	99.33
	NEW	16	100.00	100.00	99.53
Zhou et al. [8]	NEW	7	92.58	91.87	90.51
Feng [9]	NEW	7	100.00	99.44	99.18
	NEW	7	100.00	99.75	99.02
	NEW	7	100.00	100.00	99.45
Phillips et al. [10]	NEW	6	100.00	100.00	99.49
Sun [11]	NEW	14	100.00	99.56	98.63
	NEW	14	100.00	100.00	99.45
Liu [12]	NEW	7	100.00	99.62	99.02
	NEW	7	100.00	100.00	99.41
Liu [13]	NEW	16	98.64	97.12	97.02
	NEW	16	99.09	98.94	98.39
	NEW	16	99.85	99.69	98.94
	NEW	16	100.00	100.00	99.49
Yang et al. [14]	NEW	12	97.12	95.94	95.69
	NEW	12	100.00	99.69	98.98
	NEW	12	100.00	100.00	99.18
	NEW	12	100.00	100.00	99.57
Nayak et al. [15]	OLD	13	100.00	99.30	98.44
	OLD	13	100.00	100.00	99.53
Atangana [16]	NEW	6	100.00	100.00	99.53
Zhou et al. [17]	NEW	7	100.00	99.56	98.51
	NEW	7	100.00	99.69	98.55
	NEW	7	100.00	99.69	99.06
Yang [18]	NEW	12	100.00	99.69	98.43
	NEW	12	100.00	99.75	99.25
	NEW	12	100.00	100.00	99.57

(continued)

Table 10.7 (continued)

Approach	Repetition number	Feature number	DI	DII	DIII
Yang and Sun [19]	NEW	2	100.00	100.00	99.53
Sun [20]	NEW	12	99.85	98.38	97.02
	NEW	12	100.00	99.19	98.24
	NEW	12	100.00	99.31	98.12
	NEW	12	100.00	99.75	99.53
Chen [21]	NEW	5	96.52	89.31	88.78
	NEW	5	98.33	96.56	96.20
	NEW	5	97.73	93.94	92.75
	NEW	5	97.42	94.50	94.04
	NEW	5	100.00	98.19	98.08

In Table 10.6, the first column lists the author and year of publication. The second column lists the name of the employed features. The third column lists the dimension reduction (DR) technique. The fourth column lists the classifier model. The final column presents the optimization method.

In Table 10.7, the first column is a copy of the first column in Table 10.6. The second column presents the repetition number (RN).

$$RN = \begin{cases} OLD \\ NEW \end{cases}, \quad \text{if } k = \begin{cases} 5 \\ 10 \end{cases} \tag{10.4}$$

The third column shows the feature number submitted to the classifier. The final three columns show accuracy over three benchmark data sets.

10.5   Shortcomings

Two main shortcomings exist for current PBD systems:

1. The brain images in the three data sets are for instructive purposes; hence, they can be used in a textbook. This increases classification performance, leading to a near 100% accuracy. Nevertheless, this does not reflect the realistic classification results in hospitals.
2. Most PBD systems treat all types of disease as one class, that is, abnormal. This reduces the difficulty to the system, but does not reflect which type of abnormality is present. This rough classification in current PBD systems does not help physicians plan surgery.

Therefore, potential research directions include adding more brain images acquired in hospitals and increase the number of classes in current PBD systems.

References

1. Patnaik LM, Chaplot S, Jagannathan NR (2006) Classification of magnetic resonance brain images using wavelets as input to support vector machine and neural network. Biomed Signal Process Control 1(1):86–92. https://doi.org/10.1016/j.bspc.2006.05.002
2. El-Dahshan ESA, Hosny T, Salem ABM (2010) Hybrid intelligent techniques for MRI brain images classification. Digit Signal Process 20(2):433–441. https://doi.org/10.1016/j.dsp.2009.07.002
3. Wu L (2011) A hybrid method for MRI brain image classification. Expert Syst Appl 38 (8):10049–10053
4. Wu L (2012) An MR brain images classifier via principal component analysis and kernel support vector machine. Prog Electromagnet Res 130:369–388
5. Saritha M, Joseph KP, Mathew AT (2013) Classification of MRI brain images using combined wavelet entropy based spider web plots and probabilistic neural network. Pattern Recogn Lett 34(16):2151–2156. https://doi.org/10.1016/j.patrec.2013.08.017
6. Das S, Chowdhury M, Kundu MK (2013) Brain MR image classification using multiscale geometric analysis of Ripplet. Prog Electromagnet Res-Pier 137:1–17. https://doi.org/10.2528/pier13010105
7. Yang J (2015) Preclinical diagnosis of magnetic resonance (MR) brain images via discrete wavelet packet transform with Tsallis entropy and generalized eigenvalue proximal support vector machine (GEPSVM). Entropy 17(4):1795–1813. https://doi.org/10.3390/e17041795
8. Zhou X, Xu W, Sun P (2015) Detection of pathological brain in MRI scanning based on wavelet-entropy and naive Bayes classifier. In: Ortuño F, Rojas I (eds) Bioinformatics and biomedical engineering, Granada, Spain lecture notes in computer science. Springer International Publishing, pp 201–209. https://doi.org/10.1007/978-3-319-16483-0_20
9. Feng C (2015) Feed-forward neural network optimized by hybridization of PSO and ABC for abnormal brain detection. Int J Imaging Syst Technol 25(2):153–164. https://doi.org/10.1002/ima.22132
10. Phillips P, Dong Z, Yang J (2015) Pathological brain detection in magnetic resonance imaging scanning by wavelet entropy and hybridization of biogeography-based optimization and particle swarm optimization. Prog Electromagnet Res 152:41–58. https://doi.org/10.2528/PIER15040602
11. Sun P (2015) Pathological brain detection based on wavelet entropy and Hu moment invariants. Bio-Med Mater Eng 26(s1):1283–1290. https://doi.org/10.2528/PIER13121310
12. Liu A (2015) Magnetic resonance brain image classification via stationary wavelet transform and generalized eigenvalue proximal support vector machine. J Med Imaging Health Inform 5 (7):1395–1403. https://doi.org/10.1166/jmihi.2015.1542
13. Liu G (2015) Pathological brain detection in MRI scanning by wavelet packet Tsallis entropy and fuzzy support vector machine. SpringerPlus 4(1), Article ID: 716
14. Yang X, Sun P, Dong Z, Liu A, Yuan T-F (2015) Pathological brain detection by a novel image feature—fractional fourier entropy. Entropy 17(12):8278–8296. https://doi.org/10.3390/e17127877
15. Nayak DR, Dash R, Majhi B (2016) Brain MR image classification using two-dimensional discrete wavelet transform and AdaBoost with random forests. Neurocomputing 177:188–197. https://doi.org/10.1016/j.neucom.2015.11.034
16. Atangana A (2016) Application of stationary wavelet entropy in pathological brain detection. Multimed Tools Appl. https://doi.org/10.1007/s11042-016-3401-7
17. Zhou X-X, Yang J-F, Sheng H, Wei L, Yan J, Sun P (2016) Combination of stationary wavelet transform and kernel support vector machines for pathological brain detection. Simulation 92(9):827–837. https://doi.org/10.1177/0037549716629227
18. Yang M (2016) Dual-tree complex wavelet transform and twin support vector machine for pathological brain detection. Appl Sci 6(6), Article ID: 169

19. Yang JF, Sun P (2016) Magnetic resonance brain classification by a novel binary particle swarm optimization with mutation and time-varying acceleration coefficients. Biomed Eng Biomed Tech 61(4):431–441. https://doi.org/10.1515/bmt-2015-0152
20. Sun Y (2016) A multilayer perceptron based smart pathological brain detection system by fractional fourier entropy. J Med Syst 40(7), Article ID: 173. https://doi.org/10.1007/s10916-016-0525-2
21. Chen X-Q (2016) Fractal dimension estimation for developing pathological brain detection system based on Minkowski-Bouligand method. IEEE Access 4:5937–5947. https://doi.org/10.1109/ACCESS.2016.2611530

Chapter 11
Deep Learning for Cerebral Microbleed Identification

Cerebral microbleeds (CMBs) are the small foci of chronic blood products. CMBs are closely related to many diseases such as dementia, siderosis, ageing, etc. A data balance method is used for their identification, since CMB voxels in collected brain images are usually about 2000 times less common than non-CMB voxels. Two deep-learning methods: the 7-layer stacked sparse autoencoder (SAE) and the 5-layer convolutional neural network (CNN), with rank-based average pooling, are developed and tested for identifying CMB. The results show that the CNN obtains a sensitivity of 96.94%, a specificity of 97.18%, and an accuracy of 97.18%. The results of the CNN are better than those of the SAE. Both deep-learning methods are superior to four of the state-of-the-art CMB identification approaches. Besides this, experiments have showed that in the CNN, rank-based average pooling gives better results than maximum-pooling and average pooling, and that the 5-layer CNN provides better sensitivity than the 3-layer CNN and 9-layer CNN.

11.1 Cerebral Microbleeds

CMBs [1] are the foci of chronic blood products. They are closely related with glomerular filtration [2], dementia [3], cortical superficial siderosis [4], and ageing [5]. A CMB is now an obviously noticeable entity, because of the rapid development of magnetic resonance imaging (MRI), especially susceptibility weighted imaging (SWI). The hemosiderin within CMB foci is superparamagnetic, which causes significant local inhomogeneity in the magnetic field around a CMB, leading to fast decay of the MRI signal. Hence, CMB appear hypointensively in the scanned image. Nevertheless, the CMBs may be confused with vein and blood vessels.

Traditional interpretation depends on the microbleed anatomical rating scale (MARS) [6] that draws up stringent rules for classifying CMB into two types: "definite" and "possible" [7]. Nevertheless, manual interpretation is not reliable due

© Springer Nature Singapore Pte Ltd. 2018
S.-H. Wang et al., *Pathological Brain Detection*, Brain Informatics and Health,
https://doi.org/10.1007/978-981-10-4026-9_11

to high intra-observer and inter-observer variability. Visual screening is prone to either confuse CMBs with other similar issues, or simply miss small CMBs [8].

In the last decade, computer scientists have tried to solve this problem based on computer vision and image-processing techniques. Fazlollahi et al. [9] combined a multiscale mechanism and Laplacian or Gaussian approach (they abbreviated it as MSLoG). They also used random forest (RF) classifiers. Seghier et al. [10] proposed a technique called microbleed detection via automated segmentation (MIDAS). Barnes et al. [11] relied on a statistical thresholding algorithm to detect hypointensity. They then used a support vector machine (SVM) classifier to separate true CMBs from others issues. Bian et al. [12] employed a 2D fast radial symmetry transform (RST) to detect putative CMBs. Afterwards, false results were removed using features of geometry. Kuijf et al. [13] presented an RST method. Charidimou et al. [14] discussed the principles, methodologies, and rationale of CMBs and their mapping in vascular dementia. Bai et al. [15] detected CMBs in super-acute ischemic stroke patients treated with intravenous thrombolysis. Roy et al. [16] proposed a novel multiple radial symmetry transform (MRST) and RF method. Chen [17] used a leaky rectified linear unit (LReLU). Hou and Chen [18] proposed a four-layer, deep neural network (DNN) method.

Nevertheless, the detection accuracies of all the methods above are still quite low. For example: Bai's method [15] combined multimodality imaging, but they did not use a computer vision approach to increase the identification performance. Roy's method [16] obtained a sensitivity of 85.7%, which is quite high compared with human interpretation, but it did not explore the power of computer vision fully. Hou's method [19] validated that LReLU performed better than other activation functions, however, that particular study lacked theoretical analysis. Hou's method [18] showed that the DNN gave better results, but the structure of their DNN was shallow, so the potential of DNN was not explored fully.

Recently, the "deep learning" technique [20] has been proposed for machine learning. It gained significant interest and achieved remarkable achievements. The AlphaGo [21] used deep learning to beat the world champion in five-game match of Go. It was the first time that a computer had beaten a nine-dan professional player [22]. Besides this, deep learning has been successfully applied in system identification, human activity recognition [23], facial retouching detection, video tracking [24], etc.

11.2 Subjects

Ten cerebral autosomal-dominant arteriopathy, with subcortical infarcts and leukoencephalopathy (CADASIL), patients and ten healthy controls (HCs) were enrolled. We reconstructed the 3D volumetric image using Syngo MR B17 software, its size being $364 \times 448 \times 48$ pixels.

Three neuroradiologists, with over 20 years of experience, carried out manual detection of CMBs. In their analysis, they labelled "possible" and "definite" detections, which were all regarded as CMB voxels, with the others regarded as non-CMB voxels. CMB voxels are shown within the red lines in Fig. 11.1. The exclusion criteria applied two rules: (1) blood vessels were discarded by tracking through neighboring slices and (2) lesions larger than 10 mm were not considered.

(The susceptibility weighted imaging (SWI) images were obtained using a 3T SIEMENS Verio scanner on an MRC 40810 workstation. Slice number = 48; sequence = swi3d1r; flip angle = 15°; bit depth = 12; resolution = [0.5 × 0.5 × 2] mm³; slice thickness = 2 mm; echo time = 20 ms; repetition time = 28 ms; and bandwidth = 120 Hx/px.)

Fig. 11.1 Slice of a CMB. Note: *SI*, slice index

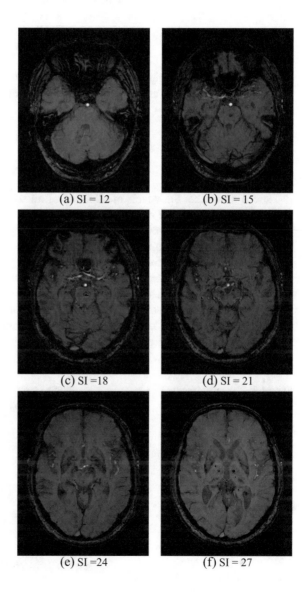

(a) SI = 12

(b) SI = 15

(c) SI = 18

(d) SI = 21

(e) SI = 24

(f) SI = 27

11.3   Data Set Generation

A sliding neighborhood processing (SNP) technique was employed to generate the input and target data sets from the 20 volumetric 3D brain images. We processed each slice of each subject. Since we know the neighborhood of a pixel p is a matrix, we vectorize this matrix to form an input sample x, then the status of the central pixel is defined as its target value y. Mathematically this is represented as:

$$x(p) = V\{N(p)\} \tag{11.1}$$

$$y(p) = \begin{cases} 1 & p \text{ is CMB voxel} \\ 0 & p \text{ is non-CMB voxel} \end{cases} \tag{11.2}$$

where N represents the neighborhood and V represents the vectorization operation. The final input data set X and target data set Y are formed by processing all voxels in set A:

$$X = \{x(p)|p \in A\} \tag{11.3}$$

$$Y = \{y(p)|p \in A\} \tag{11.4}$$

Here A represents the voxels of all slices of all subjects except the border.

In this study, we chose a window size of 61×61 pixels, namely, the voxels of the 30-pixel borders were discarded, as shown in Fig. 11.2. The window moves toward right and down so as to cover set A. Finally, we generated 68,847 CMB voxels and 113,165,073 non-CMB voxels.

The SNP technique extracts the neighborhood of a central voxel as the input of each sample, and the status of that central voxel as the target. Figure 11.3 shows nine examples of CMB voxels and nine examples of non-CMB voxels. We can observe that the 61×61 neighborhood is large enough for human interpretation, thus, the window size is considered reasonable. Recently, convolutional implementation of sliding window was proposed in OverFeat by turning the

Fig. 11.2 The relationship of window size and border width. (green represents the border area, the red rectangle represents the window, the red dot represents the central voxel, and the blue area represents set A in this slice)

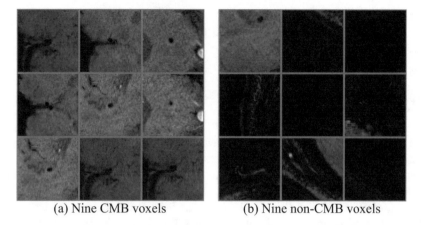

| (a) Nine CMB voxels | (b) Nine non-CMB voxels |

Fig. 11.3 Generated 61 × 61 neighborhoods of central voxels

fully-connect layer into convolution layer. Nevertheless, our intertest objects (i.e., CMB regions) in the brain image are too small revisiting Fig. 11.1. Hence, this convolutional implementation is not suitable for this task.

11.4 Autoencoder-Based Cerebral Microbleed Identification

11.4.1 Balanced Data

Imbalanced data causes severe problems to the classification, since the non-CMB voxels number 1644 times the CMB voxels. The classifier is prone to be trained nonsense as the output is 1 all the time, hence, training is not necessary. This gives the performance outlined in Table 11.1, with the sensitivity being 0%, the specificity 100%, and the accuracy 99.93%. This suggests that specificity and accuracy are not good indicators in this study. Therefore, we should focus more on the measure of sensitivity.

This imbalanced data problem arising from the area of foci of a microbleed is extremely small compared to healthy tissues. This causes an "accuracy paradox [25]," shown in Table 11.1. Many methods can solve or mitigate the imbalanced

Table 11.1 A nonsense classifier with higher accuracy

Measure	Result
Behavior	Output 1 always
Sensitivity	0%
Specificity	100.00%
Accuracy	99.93%

data problem, such as cost function–based techniques and sampling-based approaches. In this study, we used the undersampling technique to reduce the 113,165,073 samples to 68,854.

11.4.2   Autoencoder

An autoencoder (AE) is a symmetrical neural network that learns the features in an unsupervised manner. Autoencoders have been successfully applied in image reconstruction [26], image super-resolution [27], prediction [28], etc. The structure of an AE is shown in Fig. 7.4, where the encoder part is has a weight $E = [e(1), e(2), ..., e(m)]$ and a bias $B_1 = [b_1(1), b_1(2), ... b_1(m)]$, and the decoder part has a weight $D = [d(1), d(2), ..., d(m)]$ and a bias $B_2 = [b_2(1), b_2(2), ... b_2(m)]$. The encoder and decoder parts combine to make the output data $Y = [y_1, y_2, ..., y_n]$ equal to the input vector $X = [x_1, x_2, ..., x_n]$. Suppose the activation function is in logistic sigmoid form, we have:

$$a_i = \mathrm{sigm}(e(i) \times x + b_1(i)) \tag{11.5}$$

where $A = [a_1, a_2, ..., a_m]$ is the output of the hidden layer. Then, the decoding of A is carried out as:

$$y_i = \mathrm{sigm}(d(i) \times a_i + b_2(i)) \tag{11.6}$$

11.4.3   Sparse Autoencoder

To minimize the error between the input vector X and output Y, we can yield the objective function as:

$$J(E, D, B_1, B_2) = \frac{1}{2}\|Y - X\|^2 \tag{11.7}$$

From Eqs. (11.5) and (11.6), we can deduce that Y can be expressed as:

$$Y = h(X|E, D, B_1, B_2) \tag{11.8}$$

Hence, Eq. (11.7) can be revised as:

$$J(E, D, B_1, B_2) = \frac{1}{2}\|h(X|E, D, B_1, B_2) - X\|^2 \tag{11.9}$$

To avoid over-complete mapping or trivial mapping, we add one regularization term to the weight and one regularization term of a sparse constraint:

$$J(E, D, B_1, B_2) = \frac{1}{2}\|h(X|E, D, B_1, B_2) - X\|^2$$
$$+ \alpha \sum_j K(\rho, \rho_j) + \beta\| E \quad D \|_2^2 \tag{11.10}$$

where α is the weight of sparse penalty and β the regularization factor controlling the degree of weight decay. This model is called the sparse autoencoder (SAE). Here $K()$ is the Kullback–Leibler divergence defined as:

$$K(a, b) = a \times \log\frac{a}{b} + (1 - a) \times \log\frac{1 - a}{1 - b} \tag{11.11}$$

The symbol ρ represents the desired probability of being activated and ρ_j the average activation probability of the jth hidden neuron. The training procedure is performed by scaled conjugate gradient descent (SCGD) method.

11.4.4   Softmax Layer

The softmax classifier is used as the last layer in the DNN, aiming to classify the learned features from the SAE beforehand. The "softmax" is more suitable to provide an end-to-end training than "max" function. We can use "max" during the test stage. Remember that a logistic regression is a binary classifier defined as:

$$h(x|\theta) = \frac{1}{1 + \exp(-\theta^T x)} \tag{11.12}$$

where θ represents the model parameters.

In contrast, the softmax classifier uses softmax as the activation function and it can be regarded as a multinomial logistic regression with an output having k values as:

$$h(x|\theta) = \begin{bmatrix} p(y = 1|x, \theta) \\ p(y = 2|x, \theta) \\ \cdots \\ p(y = k|x, \theta) \end{bmatrix} = \frac{1}{\sum_j \exp\left(\theta_j^T x\right)} \begin{bmatrix} \exp(\theta_1^T x) \\ \exp(\theta_2^T x) \\ \cdots \\ \exp(\theta_k^T x) \end{bmatrix} \tag{11.13}$$

The values of parameter θ can be obtained by the iterative optimization algorithm on the loss function, which uses cross entropy in this study. The softmax classifier is also called multinomial logistic regression.

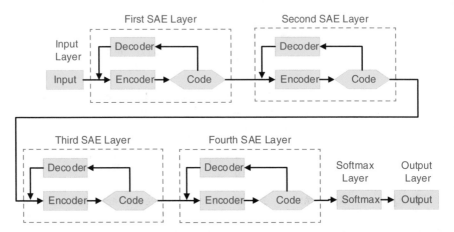

Fig. 11.4 Pipeline diagram of our stacked SAE

11.4.5 Stacked Sparse Autoencoder

The SAE was stacked to extract brain image features gradually. The feature code of each hidden layer was transmitted to the next layer, as shown in Fig. 11.4.

The structure of the proposed DNN was established. Here we create a seven-layer DNN, consisting of one input layer, four SAE layers, one softmax layer, and one output layer. The four SAE layers share the same structure, but their sizes are different. The size of each layer was selected by experience:

- The input layer had 61 * 61 = 3721 neurons.
- The first SAE layer had 1500 hidden neurons.
- The second SAE layer had 900 hidden neurons.
- The third SAE layer had 500 hidden neurons.
- The fourth SAE layer had 100 hidden neurons.
- The softmax layer had one neuron indicating a CMB voxel or non-CMB voxel.
- The output layer was directly linked to the softmax layer.

In total, we created a seven-layer SAE-DNN with a structure of 3721-1500-900-500-100-1-1. Remember that weights and biases were assigned to only the SAE and softmax layers, and not to input and output layers. For statistical analysis, 10-fold cross validation was used, and the average out-of-sample error was reported.

11.4.6 Classification Performance

The classification performance of our method over 10 runs of 10-fold cross validation is shown in Table 11.2. On average, the sensitivity was 95.13 ± 0.84%, the specificity was 93.33 ± 0.84%, and the accuracy was 94.23 ± 0.84% [29].

Table 11.2 Classification performance of our method

Run index	Sensitivity (%)	Specificity (%)	Accuracy (%)
1	94.51	92.73	93.62
2	94.78	92.98	93.88
3	94.98	93.17	94.08
4	95.68	93.90	94.79
5	94.52	92.73	93.62
6	94.29	92.47	93.38
7	94.21	92.34	93.28
8	95.56	93.70	94.63
9	96.72	94.88	95.80
10	96.10	94.31	95.21
Average	95.13 ± 0.84	93.33 ± 0.84	94.23 ± 0.84

Sensitivity was the most important measure, since it represented the ability detect CMBs from healthy controls. Specificity was less important, since misclassification of healthy people is something which can be corrected with further diagnosis.

11.5   Convolutional Neural Network–Based Cerebral Microbleed Identification

11.5.1   Cost-Sensitive Learning

Considering the data imbalance in our data set, we employed cost sensitive learning to improve the classification performance. We denote CMB voxels as the positive class (+), which is in the minority, and non-CMB voxels as the majority class (−). Assume that $C(i, j)$ is the cost of predicting the positive example class i to the negative example class j. The cost matrix is displayed in Table 11.3.

If we assume that there is no cost for correct classifications, then the cost ratio can be expresses as:

$$\text{Cost ratio} = \frac{C(-, +)}{C(+, -)} \tag{11.14}$$

Table 11.3 Cost matrix

Actual class	Predicted class	
	CMB	Non-CMB
CMB	$C(+, +)$	$C(-, +)$
Non-CMB	$C(+, -)$	$C(-, -)$

Then, the minimum misclassification cost can be expressed as:

$$\text{Total Cost} = C(-, +) \times N_{\text{FN}} + C(+, -) \times N_{\text{FP}} \qquad (11.15)$$

where N_{FN} and N_{FP} stand for the number of the false positive and false negative samples, respectively.

11.5.2   Structure of the Convolutional Neural Network

The CNN is shift covariant in detection, therefore, we used it for CMB detection. It is composed of multiple layers to implement different functions: convolution layers, pooling layers, rectified linear unit (ReLU) layers, and fully connected layers. Each layer has learnable parameters and carries out a linear transformation followed by a nonlinear transformation, which is utilized to accelerate the training process. Figure 11.5 shows the structure of the CNN. Based on the training algorithm, the CNN classifies input image sliding as a CMB or non-CMB.

11.5.3   Convolution Layer and Rectified Linear Unit Layer

The operation on two functions of a real-valued argument is called convolution. Figure 11.6 shows an example of the convolution for the first four steps applied in the spatial domain.

In the convolution layer, a set of linear activation functions is generated via convolutions in parallel. Afterwards, there is a nonlinear activation layer to implement a nonlinear transformation.

The most common functions used for the output of the convolution layer for nonlinear mapping include: hyperbolic tangent activation, softmax activation, rectified linear unit activation, etc. For the CNN, we selected the ReLU as the activation function. Mathematically, ReLU can be expressed as follows.

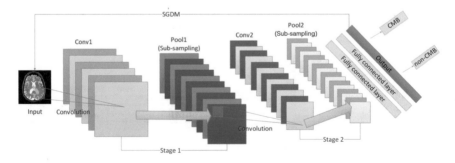

Fig. 11.5 Structure of the CNN

Fig. 11.6 Sample of convolution

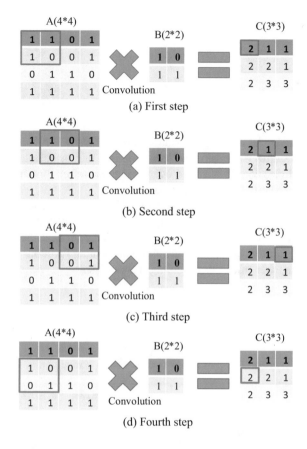

(a) First step

(b) Second step

(c) Third step

(d) Fourth step

Suppose the inputs to a neuron are x, then:

$$f(x) = \max(0, x) \qquad (11.16)$$

The ReLU was first introduced by Hahnloser et al. [30] for a dynamic network. For convolution networks, ReLU is more effective than the logistic sigmoid function, and more practical than the hyperbolic tangent. For these reasons, the ReLU has become the most popular activation function for the CNN.

11.5.4 Pooling Layer

Using all the features obtained from the convolution layer could create a high burden on classification computations. Here, we take an image of size 61 * 61 as an example, and suppose we have learned 400 features over the 8 * 8 inputs. We can get an output of size (61 − 8 + 1) * (61 − 8 + 1) = 2916 from the convolution

Fig. 11.7 Max pooling

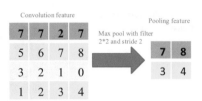

layer. As we had 400 features, this will result in a vector of 2916 * 400 = 1166,400 features for a sample. Now, over one million features for a classifier may cause a dimension disaster and over-fitting. Therefore, pooling is essential for the CNN to reduce the feature numbers.

The pooling function essentially replaces the output of a net with a summary statistic of the nearby outputs at a certain location. Pooling technology can make less sensitive activations in the pooled map than the original feature map.

Since it is possible that different pooling functions perform differently, we used a number of different pooling technologies.

11.5.4.1   Max Pooling

Max pooling [31]. In max pooling, the matrix $u(x, y)$ is applied to the convolution features. The maximum output within a rectangular neighborhood is recorded:

$$M_j = \max_{N \times N}\left(M_i^{n \times n} u(n, n)\right) \tag{11.17}$$

Here, M stands for the inputs of the pooling layer and $M_i^{n \times n}$ is a sub-matrix of M. Figure 11.7 shows an example of max pooling.

11.5.4.2   Average Pooling

Average pooling. The average pooling function takes an average over the inputs. Both methods obtain a feature map with a lower resolution.

11.5.4.3   Rank-Based Average Pooling

Rank-based average pooling [32]. Average pooling considers the average operation for near-zero negative activations. Average pooling may downplay higher activation values and cause loss of discriminative information. Similarly, non-maximum activations are completely discarded in max pooling, which can cause loss of information. Rank-based average pooling (RAP) can overcome these problems of the loss of useful information caused by the max pooling and average pooling [33]. The output of RAP can be expressed as:

$$S_j = \frac{1}{t} \sum_{i \in R_j, r_i < t} a_i \qquad (11.18)$$

where t stands for the rank threshold, which determines the types of activations involved in averaging; R is the pooling region j in feature maps; t represents the index of each activation within it; and s_j and a_i stand for the rank of activation i and the value of activation i, respectively. Here, if $t = 1$, the process becomes max pooling. Therefore, t should be set properly to be certain that RAP can gain a good trade-off between average pooling and max pooling. Using the median value of t can remove negative or low value activations while keeping high-response activations.

11.5.5 Training Method and Network Structure

CNN training was implemented on the NVIDIA GeForce GTX 1050 platform, with a computer capability of 6.1, clock rate of 1455 MHz, and Intel® Core™ i5 multiprocessors. We employed stochastic gradient descent with momentum (SGDM), which utilized the full training set to compute the next update of parameters at each iteration. This procedure tended to cover local optima well. Traditionally, it is intractable, on a single machine, to compute the cost and gradient for the whole training set in case the data set is too big to fit in the main memory. Furthermore, batch optimization methods do not give an easy way to incorporate new data in an "online" setting. Stochastic gradient descent (SGD) addressed these two problems. The standard gradient descent algorithm updates the parameter θ of the objective function $f(\theta)$ as:

$$\theta = \theta - \alpha \nabla_\theta E[f(\theta)] \qquad (11.20)$$

in which α is the learning rate.

However, standard SGD tends to oscillate across the narrow ravine, especially in cases where the objective has the form of a long shallow ravine, which leads to optimum and steep walks on the sides. Thus, momentum is adopted to push the objective more quickly along the shallow ravine.

The minibatch size was set at 128 in our experiments. The initial learning rate was set at 0.01, and was decreased by factor of 10 every 10 epochs. The momentum was set to 0.9. We set the maximum number of epochs at 30. The loss function was set as the cross entropy.

Table 11.4 gives details of the CNN we designed with five layers. The pooling method used was RAP. The number of filters used for the convolution was 40, 80, 120, 160, and 240 respectively for each layer. N.B., modern CNNs may replace pooling with strided convolution and replace FCL with global average pooling, providing an all convolutional net. In this book, we only consider traditional CNNs. Dropout layers are usually put before FCL to help regularization; nevertheless, our two FCL layers do not have too many parameters, and hence we do not use dropout technique.

Table 11.4 Structure of the designed CNN

Index	Layer	Filter	Number of filters	Stride	Padding	Weights	Bias	Activation
1	Image input layer							$61 \times 61 \times 1$
2	Conv + ReLU	3×3	40	[3 3]	[1 1]	$3 \times 3 \times 1 \times 40$	$1 \times 1 \times 40$	$21 \times 21 \times 40$
3	Pooling	3×3		[1 1]	[1 1]			$21 \times 21 \times 40$
4	Conv + ReLU	5×5	80	[2 2]	[0 0]	$5 \times 5 \times 40 \times 80$	$1 \times 1 \times 80$	$9 \times 9 \times 80$
5	Pooling	3×3		[1 1]	[1 1]			$9 \times 9 \times 80$
6	Conv + ReLU	3×3	120	[1 1]	[1 1]	$3 \times 3 \times 80 \times 120$	$1 \times 1 \times 120$	$9 \times 9 \times 120$
7	Pooling	3×3		[1 1]	[1 1]			$9 \times 9 \times 120$
8	Conv + ReLU	3×3	160	[1 1]	[1 1]	$3 \times 3 \times 120 \times 160$	$1 \times 1 \times 160$	$9 \times 9 \times 160$
9	Pooling	3×3		[1 1]	[1 1]			$9 \times 9 \times 160$
10	Conv + ReLU	3×3	240	[1 1]	[1 1]	$3 \times 3 \times 160 \times 240$	$1 \times 1 \times 240$	$9 \times 9 \times 240$
11	Pooling	3×3		[1 1]	[1 1]			$9 \times 9 \times 240$
12	FCL					$100 \times 19{,}440$	100×1	
13	FCL					2×100	2×1	

Conv convolution; *FCL* fully connected layer

11.5.6 Classification Result

Based on the above designed structure with RAP, we get an average classification accuracy of 97.18%. The training accuracy improved to 90% when the iteration number was $4 * 10^6$. The training loss showed a sharp decrease between iteration number $3 * 10^6$ and $6 * 10^6$, the decrease then slowed until the best training loss was reached (Figs. 11.8 and 11.9).

From Table 11.5, we can see that the designed CNN correctly detected 33,632 CMB voxels and 27,667,564 non-CMB voxels on its first run. Table 11.6 shows the results for 10 runs. The average sensitivity across these runs was 96.94%, the average specificity was 97.18%, and the average accuracy was 97.18%. The standard deviations of the sensitivity, specificity, and accuracy, based on the 10 runs, are 0.90687, 0.70, and 0.70, respectively.

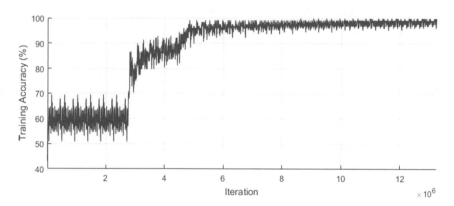

Fig. 11.8 Training accuracy

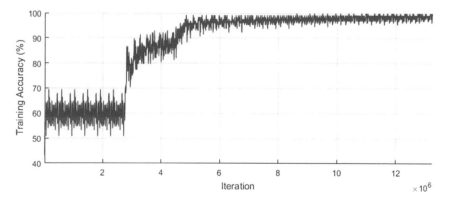

Fig. 11.9 Training loss

Table 11.5 The confusion matrix of CMB detection for the first run

Actual class	Predicted class	
	CMB (34,424)	Non-CMB (28,281,268)
CMB	33,632	613,704
Non-CMB	792	27,667,564

Table 11.6 Specificity, sensitivity, and accuracy of the designed CNN for 10 runs

Measurements	Sensitivity (%)	Specificity (%)	Accuracy (%)
1st run	97.70	97.83	97.83
2nd run	96.89	96.91	96.91
3rd run	97.58	97.56	97.56
4th run	96.53	96.58	96.58
5th run	97.71	97.75	97.75
6th run	96.83	97.12	97.12
7th run	95.27	96.74	96.74
8th run	95.82	95.93	95.93
9th run	96.85	97.10	97.10
10th run	98.20	98.32	98.32
Std	0.90687	0.70	0.70
Mean	96.94	97.18	97.18

11.5.7   Convolutional Neural Network with Different Structures

We designed a 5-conv layer CNN for CMB detection. Research shows that the layer number has a strong relation to the performance. Therefore, we compare here the 5-conv layer CNN with the 3-conv layer CNN and 9-conv layer CNN [34]. The results are shown in Table 11.7; we find that the 5-conv layer CNN has the best performance. It achieved a sensitivity of 96.94%, specificity of 97.18%, and an accuracy of 97.18%.

In this chapter, we proposed using the CNN for CMB classification. In order to do this, we worked with 10 CADASIL patients. We first employed the SNP technique to generate input images. Considering the data imbalance of the CMB voxels and non-CMB voxels, cost ratio was used. Finally, we used the CNN for CMB voxel detection. Sensitivity, specificity, and accuracy were employed as the

Table 11.7 CNN with different numbers of structures

	Sensitivity (%)	Specificity (%)	Accuracy (%)
CNN (5-conv layer)	96.94	97.18	97.18
CNN (3-conv layer)	96.83	96.85	96.85
CNN (9-conv layer)	96.89	97.53	97.53

measurements. The 5-conv layer CNN achieved a sensitivity of 96.94%, a specificity of 97.18% and an accuracy of 97.18%. Due to the large number of non-CMB voxels, the specificity was nearly approximate to accuracy. However, the main purpose of this research was to detect CMB voxels, Therefore, sensitivity was more important than the other two measurements. In order to prove the efficiency of the designed structure, we compared CNNs with different layers, including a 3-conv layer CNN and a 9-conv layer CNN (Table 11.7). In the future, we may try to use the shortcut concept in ResNet, to help build a deeper convolutional neural network.

11.5.8 Pooling Method Comparison

Based on the above designed 5-conv layer CNN structures, we compared different pooling technologies including max pooling, average pooling, and RAP, for an average of 10 runs. The results of the different pooling methods are given in Table 11.8.

As we can see from Table 11.8, the RAP method performed better than max pooling and average pooling. This is because RAP kept higher activation values which are thrown out by the average operation of average pooling and the non-maximum activations, which are thrown out by max pooling.

11.6 Comparison with State-of-the-Art Approaches

Finally, we compare the 7-layer SAE-DNN method in Sect. 11.4 and 5-conv layer CNN method in Sect. 11.5 with MRST + RF [16], LReLU [17], the 4-layer DNN [18], and WE + NBC [35]. The comparison results in Table 11.9 show that the proposed 5-conv layer CNN method and proposed 7-layer SAE give better results than state-of-the-art approaches.

Table 11.8 Comparison of different pooling technologies

	Max pooling	Average pooling	RAP (proposed)
Accuracy (%)	96.83	97.02	97.18

Table 11.9 Comparison of voxel-based identification

Method	Sensitivity (%)	Specificity (%)	Accuracy (%)
MRST + RF [16]	85.7	**99.5**	~
LReLU [17]	93.05	93.06	93.06
4-layer DNN [18]	93.40	93.05	93.23
WE + NBC [35]	76.90 ± 1.81	76.91 ± 1.58	76.90 ± 1.67
7-layer SAE (proposed)	95.13	93.33	94.23
5-conv layer CNN (proposed)	**96.94**	97.18	**97.18**

The MRST + RF [16] method gives the highest specificity, which is not an important measure in terms of diagnosis. In clinical conditions, sensitivity (i.e., to identify a CMB voxel) is the most important measure. Low specificity (i.e., to identify a non-CMB voxel) can be double-checked by human neuroradiologists. In all, CNN performs better than SAE in this application.

11.7 Future Direction

Scholars produced some successful detection systems (such as the Alzheimer's disease (AD) detection system) prior to starting to develop a PBD system. Can the AD detection system help us generate a PBD system? This question can resolved by considering the "transfer learning" technique, which is based on the idea that it would be easier to learn to speak Japanese having already learned to speak Chinese. Transfer learning can apply knowledge gained while developing the AD detection system, to the related problem of generating a PBD system.

Users may have a small numbers of labeled brain images and a large numbers of unlabeled brain images. When creating PBD systems, users usually discard the unlabeled brain images and merely make use of the labeled brain images. Nevertheless, scholars have found unlabeled data used with labeled data, can produce significant improvements in PBD [36]. Semi-supervised learning (SSL) is a mixture of unsupervised learning and supervised learning. It makes full use of both labeled data and unlabeled data. Therefore, the SSL technique may be practical in PBD situations.

References

1. Romero JR, Preis SR, Beiser AS, DeCarli C, Lee DY, Viswanathan A, Benjamin EJ, Fontes J, Au R, Pikula A, Wang J, Kase CS, Wolf PA, Irrizary MC, Seshadri S (2012) Lipoprotein phospholipase A2 and cerebral microbleeds in the framingham heart study. Stroke 43(11):3091–3094. https://doi.org/10.1161/strokeaha.112.656744
2. Liu YY, Lv P, Jin HQ, Cui W, Niu CG, Zhao MM, Fan CH, Teng YM, Pan B, Peng Q, Luo JJ, Zheng LM, Huang YN (2016) Association between low estimated glomerular filtration rate and risk of cerebral small-vessel diseases: a meta-analysis. J Stroke Cerebrovasc Dis 25(3):710–716. https://doi.org/10.1016/j.jstrokecerebrovasdis.2015.11.016
3. Shams S, Martola J, Granberg T, Li X, Shams M, Fereshtehnejad SM, Cavallin L, Aspelin P, Kristoffersen-Wiberg M, Wahlund LO (2015) Cerebral microbleeds: different prevalence, topography, and risk factors depending on dementia diagnosis—the Karolinska imaging dementia study. Am J Neuroradiol 36(4):661–666. https://doi.org/10.3174/ajnr.A4176
4. Inoue Y, Nakajima M, Uetani H, Hirai T, Ueda M, Kitajima M, Utsunomiya D, Watanabe M, Hashimoto M, Ikeda M, Yamashita Y, Ando Y (2016) Diagnostic significance of cortical superficial siderosis for Alzheimer disease in patients with cognitive impairment. Am J Neuroradiol 37(2):223–227. https://doi.org/10.3174/ajnr.A4496
5. Del Brutto OH, Mera RM, Ha JE, Del Brutto VJ, Castillo PR, Zambrano M, Gillman J (2016) Oily   fish   consumption   is   inversely   correlated   with   cerebral   microbleeds   in

community-dwelling older adults: results from the Atahualpa project. Aging Clin Exp Res 28(4):737–743. https://doi.org/10.1007/s40520-015-0473-6

6. Gregoire SM, Chaudhary UJ, Brown MM, Yousry TA, Kallis C, Jager HR, Werring DJ (2009) The microbleed anatomical rating scale (MARS): reliability of a tool to map brain microbleeds. Neurology 73(21):1759–1766. https://doi.org/10.1212/WNL.0b013e3181c34a7d

7. Banerjee G, Wahab KW, Gregoire SM, Jichi F, Charidimou A, Jager HR, Rantell K, Werring DJ (2016) Impaired renal function is related to deep and mixed, but not strictly lobar cerebral microbleeds in patients with ischaemic stroke and TIA. J Neurol 263(4):760–764. https://doi.org/10.1007/s00415-016-8040-4

8. Peng Q, Sun W, Liu WH, Liu R, Huang YN (2016) Longitudinal relationship between chronic kidney disease and distribution of cerebral microbleeds in patients with ischemic stroke. J Neurol Sci 362:1–6. https://doi.org/10.1016/j.jns.2016.01.015

9. Fazlollahi A, Meriaudeau F, Giancardo L, Villemagne VL, Rowe CC, Yates P, Salvado O, Bourgeat P (2015) Computer-aided detection of cerebral microbleeds in susceptibility-weighted imaging. Comput Med Imaging Graph 46:269–276. https://doi.org/10.1016/j.compmedimag.2015.10.001

10. Seghier ML, Kolanko MA, Leff AP, Jager HR, Gregoire SM, Werring DJ (2011) Microbleed detection using automated segmentation (MIDAS): a new method applicable to standard clinical MR images. Plos One 6(3), Article ID: e17547. https://doi.org/10.1371/journal.pone.0017547

11. Barnes SRS, Haacke EM, Ayaz M, Boikov AS, Kirsch W, Kido D (2011) Semiautomated detection of cerebral microbleeds in magnetic resonance images. Magn Reson Imaging 29(6):844–852. https://doi.org/10.1016/j.mri.2011.02.028

12. Bian W, Hess CP, Chang SM, Nelson SJ, Lupo JM (2013) Computer-aided detection of radiation-induced cerebral microbleeds on susceptibility-weighted MR images. Neuroimage-Clinical 2:282–290. https://doi.org/10.1016/j.nicl.2013.01.012

13. Kuijf HJ, de Bresser J, Geerlings MI, Conijn MMA, Viergever MA, Biessels GJ, Vincken KL (2012) Efficient detection of cerebral microbleeds on 7.0 T MR images using the radial symmetry transform. Neuroimage 59(3):2266–2273. https://doi.org/10.1016/j.neuroimage.2011.09.061

14. Charidimou A, Jager HR, Werring DJ (2012) Cerebral microbleed detection and mapping: principles, methodological aspects and rationale in vascular dementia. Exp Gerontol 47(11):843–852. https://doi.org/10.1016/j.exger.2012.06.008

15. Bai QK, Zhao ZG, Sui HJ, Xie XH, Chen J, Yang J, Zhang L (2013) Susceptibility-weighted imaging for cerebral microbleed detection in super-acute ischemic stroke patients treated with intravenous thrombolysis. Neurol Res 35(6):586–593. https://doi.org/10.1179/1743132813y.0000000179

16. Roy S, Jog A, Magrath E, Butman JA, Pham DL (2015) Cerebral microbleed segmentation from susceptibility weighted images. In: Proceedings of SPIE, vol 9413, Article ID: 94131E. https://doi.org/10.1117/12.2082237

17. Chen Y (2016) Voxelwise detection of cerebral microbleed in CADASIL patients by leaky rectified linear unit and early stopping: A class-imbalanced susceptibility-weighted imaging data study. Multimed Tools Appl. https://doi.org/10.1007/s11042-017-4383-9

18. Hou X-X, Chen H (2016) Sparse autoencoder based deep neural network for voxelwise detection of cerebral microbleed. In: 22nd International conference on parallel and distributed systems, Wuhan, China. IEEE, pp 34–37

19. Hou X-X (2017) Voxelwise detection of cerebral microbleed in CADASIL patients by leaky rectified linear unit and early stopping. Multimed Tools Appl. https://doi.org/10.1007/s11042-017-4383-9

20. Erfani SM, Rajasegarar S, Karunasekera S, Leckie C (2016) High-dimensional and large-scale anomaly detection using a linear one-class SVM with deep learning. Pattern Recogn 58:121–134. https://doi.org/10.1016/j.patcog.2016.03.028

21. Chen JX (2016) The evolution of computing: AlphaGo. Comput Sci Eng 18(4):4–7

22. Silver D, Huang A, Maddison CJ, Guez A, Sifre L, van den Driessche G, Schrittwieser J, Antonoglou I, Panneershelvam V, Lanctot M, Dieleman S, Grewe D, Nham J, Kalchbrenner N, Sutskever I, Lillicrap T, Leach M, Kavukcuoglu K, Graepel T, Hassabis D (2016) Mastering the game of Go with deep neural networks and tree search. Nature 529(7587):484–489. https://doi.org/10.1038/nature16961

23. Ronao CA, Cho SB (2016) Human activity recognition with smartphone sensors using deep learning neural networks. Expert Syst Appl 59:235–244. https://doi.org/10.1016/j.eswa.2016.04.032

24. Xue HY, Liu Y, Cai D, He XF (2016) Tracking people in RGBD videos using deep learning and motion clues. Neurocomputing 204:70–76. https://doi.org/10.1016/j.neucom.2015.06.112

25. Valverde-Albacete FJ, Pelaez-Moreno C (2014) 100% Classification Accuracy considered harmful: the normalized information transfer factor explains the accuracy paradox. Plos One 9 (1), Article ID: e84217. https://doi.org/10.1371/journal.pone.0084217

26. Mehta J, Majumdar A (2017) RODEO: robust DE-aliasing autoencOder for real-time medical image reconstruction. Pattern Recogn 63:499–510. https://doi.org/10.1016/j.patcog.2016.09.022

27. Zeng K, Yu J, Wang RX, Li CH, Tao DC (2017) Coupled deep autoencoder for single image super-resolution. IEEE Trans Cybern 47(1):27–37. https://doi.org/10.1109/tcyb.2015.2501373

28. Saha M, Mitra P, Nanjundiah RS (2016) Autoencoder-based identification of predictors of Indian monsoon. Meteorol Atmos Phys 128(5):613–628. https://doi.org/10.1007/s00703-016-0431-7

29. Chen H (2017) Seven-layer deep neural network based on sparse autoencoder for voxelwise detection of cerebral microbleed. Multimed Tools Appl. https://doi.org/10.1007/s11042-017-4554-8

30. Hahnloser RHR, Sarpeshkar R, Mahowald MA, Douglas RJ, Seung HS (2000) Correction: Digital selection and analogue amplification coexist in acortex-inspired silicon circuit. Nature 405(6789):947–951

31. Masci J, Giusti A, Dan C, Fricout G, Schmidhuber J (2014) A fast learning algorithm for image segmentation with max-pooling convolutional networks. In: IEEE international conference on image processing, pp 2713–2717

32. Fernando B, Gavves E, Oramas J, Ghodrati A, Tuytelaars T (2017) Rank pooling for action recognition. IEEE Trans Pattern Anal Mach Intell 39(4):773–787. https://ieeexplore.ieee.org/document/7458903/

33. Shi ZL, Ye YD, Wu YP (2016) Rank-based pooling for deep convolutional neural networks. Neural Netw 83:21–31. https://doi.org/10.1016/j.neunet.2016.07.003

34. Jiang Y, Hou X, Cheng H, Du S (2017) Cerebral micro-bleed detection based on the convolution neural network with rank based average pooling. IEEE Access 5:16576–16583. https://doi.org/10.1109/ACCESS.2017.2736558

35. Gagnon B (2017) Cerebral microbleed detection by wavelet entropy and naive Bayes classifier. Adv Biol Sci Res 4:505–510

36. Johnson DM, Xiong CM, Corso JJ (2016) Semi-supervised nonlinear distance metric learning via forests of max-margin cluster hierarchies. IEEE Trans Knowl Data Eng 28(4):1035–1046. https://doi.org/10.1109/tkde.2015.2507130

Index

A
Activation function, 137
  logistic sigmoid, 137
  rectified linear unit, 137
    leaky ReLU, 137
Ant colony optimization, 168
  pheromone evaporation, 170
Artificial immune system, 158
  clonal selection algorithm, 158
  dendritic cell algorithm, 158
  immune network algorithm, 158
  negative selection algorithm, 158
Antigen, 156
Autoencoder, 196
  softmax, 197
  sparse autoencoder, 197
  stack, 197

B
Back-propagation, 149
  adaptive BP, 149
  momentum BP, 149
Bayes error rate, 125
Biogeography-based optimization, 171
  habitat suitability index, 171
  suitability index variable, 171
Blood oxygen level dependent, 22
Brain disease, 2
  brain tumor, 3
  cerebral microbleeding, 191
  cerebrovascular disease, 3
    transient ischemic attac, 5
  inflammatory disease, 5
    Creutzfeldt–Jakob disease, 6
    rabies, 6

neoplastic disease, 3
  neurodegeneration, 3
    Alzheimer's disease, 3
Brain segmentation, 21
  cerebrospinal fluid, 21
  gray matter, 21
  white matter, 21

C
CADASIL, 192, 206
CNN, 200
  convolution, 200
  fully connected layer, 204
  pooling layer, 201
  ReLU layer, 200
Computer-aided diagnosis, 7
Cost sensitive learning, 199
Cross entropy, 197, 203
Cross validation, 180
  k-fold cross validation, 181
  leave-one-out cross validation, 181
  leave-p-out cross validation, 181
  Monte Carlo cross validation, 183
Cumulative distribution function, 40

D
Decision tree, 122
  C4.5, 123
  classification and regression tree, 123
  ID3, 123
  random forest, 124
Dimensionality reduction, 105
Discrete Fourier transform, 56
  discrete cosine transform, 56
  discrete sine transform, 56

© Springer Nature Singapore Pte Ltd. 2018
S.-H. Wang et al., *Pathological Brain Detection*, Brain Informatics and Health,
https://doi.org/10.1007/978-981-10-4026-9